Consensus Conference on the Management
of Cystic Fibrosis

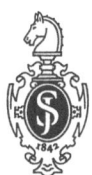

BASF Pharma, SMG/Pankreas

Consensus Conference on the Management of Cystic Fibrosis

Paris, June 3rd, 1994

With 18 Figures

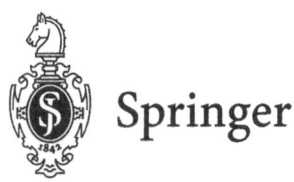 Springer

Springer-Verlag GmbH & Co. KG
Science Communication
Editing Dept. for Medicine
Priv.-Doz. Dr. B. Fruhstorfer, Dr. A. Heinz,
D. Berger, U. Hilpert, K. Kupfer, Heidelberg
Coedited by Dr. Drev R. Chadha, Wassenaar

ISBN-13:978-3-540-58766-8   e-ISBN-13:978-3-642-79444-5
ISBN: 10.1007/978-3-642-79444-5

Layout and Production Supervision: W. Bischoff, Heidelberg

16 / 3130 – 5 4 3 2 1 0 – Printed on acid-free paper

Prof. Dr. M. Antonelli
Cystic Fibrosis Center
Department of Pediatrics
University of Rome
„La Sapienza"
Viale Regina Elena 324
00161 Rome
Italy

Prof. Dr. N. Brousse
Necker-Enfants
Malades Hospital
Service Hematologie
149, Rue de Sevres
75015 Paris
France

Prof. Dr. J.A. Dodge
The Queen´s
University of Belfast
Grosvenor Road
Belfast BT12 6BJ
Northern Ireland

Prof. Dr. R. Fink
Department
of Pulmonary Medicine
Children´s National
Medical Center
11 Michigan Avenue N.W.
Washington, D.C. 20010
USA

Prof. Dr. G. Lenoir
Necker-Enfants
Malades Hospital
Clinique Robert Debré
149, Rue de Sevres
75015 Paris
France

Dr. J. Littlewood
Cystic Fibrosis Unit
St. James University
Hospital Trust
Beckett Street
Leeds LS9 7TF
UK

Prof. Dr. J.D. Lloyd-Still
Cystic Fibrosis Center
Children´s Memorial Hospital
2300 Children´s Parkway
Chicago IL 60614
USA

PD Dr. med. H.-G. Posselt
Klinikum der Johann Wolfgang
Goethe-Universität
Theodor-Stern-Kai 7
60596 Frankfurt

Dr. L. Romano
Department of Pediatrics and
CF Center
G. Gaslini Institute
Largo Gaslini, 5
16147 Genova
Italy

Dr. R. I. Smyth
Royal Liverpool
Children´s Hospital
Alder Hey
Liverpool L12 2AP
UK

Dr. C. J. Taylor
Department of Pediatrics
University of Sheffield
Sheffield S10 2TH
UK

Contents

Opening Remarks

J.A. Dodge, Belfast

The purpose of this meeting is to see what consensus there is about how we use pancreatic enzymes in cystic fibrosis. Enzyme preparations have been available for many years, and they have improved perhaps to the point where their effectiveness and dosage possibilities have gone ahead of our clinical understanding. Inevitably it was knowledge that colonic strictures had occurred in some children who were taking pancreatic enzymes, and the suggestion of a possible link between the two, that has brought this whole issue to our attention. So we meet today with the object of exploring how enzyme preparations are used in different European countries. Our discussion will be informed by a knowledge of possible complications but will not revolve around that.

It is very interesting to compare the attitudes and the regulatory managements of different countries. In the US pancreatic enzymes are regarded not as drugs, but as digestive aids, and until recently they did not need Food and Drug Administration approval. In other countries, however, they are treated as pharmacological agents. In reality the view that they are simply natural products that relate to digestion is probably not more tenable than saying that digoxin is simply digitalis leaf that has been packaged. The concentration and purification of pancreatic enzymes has been improved greatly, but still they are a very crude biological substance. The potential variability of the product, which makes it quite distinct from many drugs which can be precisely measured and dosed and will be totally consistent from one batch to another, is perhaps another area for discussion.

How do we handle these substances? We now have the technology to make them very potent, but perhaps we do not yet - at least for the high-strength products - have the experience to know their proper place in the management of patients.

Now it gives me pleasure to ask my Co-Chairman to present the results of a questionnaire which he has coordinated for the CF centres in Germany.

Presentation on the Questionnaire in CF Centres in Germany

H.-G. Posselt, Frankfurt

We have about 260 CF patients under regular care in Frankfurt. Soon after the first publication in The Lancet we sent a questionnaire to the German CF centres with the following questions:

1. How many CF patients have you cared for on a regular basis since 1985 (including those who died)?
2. How many of these patients were treated with pancreatic enzymes such as Creon 25000 or Panzytrat 20000 or 40000?
3. How many episodes of distal intestinal obstruction syndrome (DIOS) requiring special treatment did you observe in these patients?
4. How many of the DIOS patients needed surgical intervention?
5. How many of the operated DIOS patients underwent bowel resection?
6. In how many cases of the operated patients was the resected specimen available for further investigation?
7. How many patients in your care required laparotomy because of intestinal strictures (excluding neonates)?

Results of a questionnaire - German CF centres

○ Number of Germany CF centres questionnaire sent to	71
○ Number of answers available for evaluation	60
○ Total number of treated patients in these centres	3205
○ Answers available for patients treated with high-lipase preparations (%)	57
○ Answers available for analysis of the individual (%)	54
○ Number of patients with DIOS requiring specific medication	219
○ Number of patients with DIOS requiring surgical intervention	11
○ Number of operated patients needing intestinal resection	4
○ Number of patients with intestinal resections caused by indications other than DIOS	4
○ Number of resected specimens available for further histopathological evaluation	7

| CF Centres | n patients | % patients with HL prep. | Pancreatic enzyme supplementation dosage-regimen available: n =2782 patients. Lipase units/kg body weight/die | | | | | |
			0	< 5000	5000 –10000	10000 –20000	20000 –50000	<50000
60	3205	1619 52.4%	100 3.6%	939 33.8%	922 33.1%	623 22.4%	175 6.3%	23 0.8%
Range of individual dosage in the different out patients depts.			0 to 10.4%	1.3% to 94%	5.5% to 88.2%	3.0% to 97%	0 to 50%	0 to 7.1%

Fig. 1. Colonic strictures in CF-Results of questionnaire III – German CF-Centres

Seven histopathological specimens is a very small number and I think it is a big problem that we have no knowledge of normal intestinal histopathology in CF patients. The most important thing at the present time is that no patient was detected with strictures of the intestine needing surgical treatment.

To the next part of the questionnaire, how is pancreatic enzyme supplementation practised in the CF centres in Germany? We have answers from 60 centres, with 3205 patients under regular care. We have exact data about the individual dosage for only 2782 patients. We grouped patients according to the supplementation they received: none, up to 5000, 5000-10 000, 10 000-20 000, 20 000-50 000, and more than 50 000 units lipase/kg body weight/day.

As seen in Fig.1 only 7% were on dosages above 20 000 units lipase/kg body weight. However, there are very big differences between the different centres in specific dosages. The data from the Frankfurt centre from 251 patients are shown in Fig.2.

Surprisingly, the patients on the higher dosages are the younger ones. I think there is no good explanation why the smaller

Fig. 2. Pancreatic enzyme supplementation in CF (Outpatients, Frankfurt am Main, 1994)

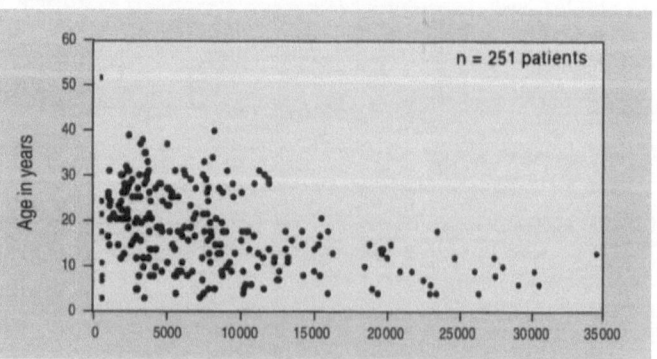

batients have this high dosage, and we need to clarify this. We have to check whether the parents increase the dosage because the stool appearance was not satisfactory.

Patients who developed strictures were taking very high doses. Many were taking more than 20 000 units/kg body weight daily. In Germany we use lower doses of lipase, and this might be why we have had no patients with strictures.

The Management of Cystic Fibrosis With Enzymes in France

G. Lenoir, C. Silly, N. Brousse, J.P. Cezard, J. Navarro, Paris

The management of pancreatic insufficiency in cystic fibrosis is still a problem in some cases, but several major concepts have to be considered:

1. Undernutrition is an important factor adversely affecting survival in CF.
2. Pancreatic enzyme extracts have been used for several decades to decrease maldigestion of nutrients and enteric coated microspheres have been a major advance in optimizing absorption overall.
3. The aim of the management of CF patients is to fully correct not only maldigestion or malabsorption but malnutrition at all as Dr. Durie clearly demonstrated at the 19th CF conference in Paris.

Physiology

Secretion of the exocrine pancreas has a good influence on absorption of nutrients and in maintaining duodenal intraluminal pH. In fact, the pancreas secretes more protein/g of tissue than any other organ. More than 85% of this protein content is made up of enzymes or proenzymes (Table 1). Everybody knows that lipase does not summarize the pancreatic secretions.

Table 1. Some pancreatic enzymes

Proteolytic enzymes

Endopeptidases	Exopeptidases
Trypsin	Carboxypeptidase A
Chymotrypsin	Carboxypeptidase B
Elastase	
Kallikrein	

Nonproteolytic enzymes
Lipase
Colipase
Phospholipase A_1, A_2
Nonspecific carboxyl esterase
Amylase
Nucleases

Pharmacology

Standardized pancreatic enzyme products obtained by freeze drying have been available in France since 1969. For the first time in the field of animal extracts it was a manufactured formulated product. However, the conventional Eurobiol ® pow—der cannot be regarded as therapeutically and pharmaceutically equivalent to the other classic preparations of pancreatic enzyme.

In 1988 Alipase® and Créon® became available commercially. These enteric-coated formulations may not be therapeutically equivalent because of differences in enzyme content and the dissolution of their enteric coatings. In 1989 the first enteric-coated high-strength product, Eurobiol 25000, was launched. It contents 25000 units of lipase, 22500 amylase and 1250 protease.

Some studies have indicated that there is no clinical difference between the microsphere preparations, but overall their superiority over conventional enzyme preparations is firmly established especially with regard to improvement in steatorrhea and lipid absorption (+ 10%).

The advantages of enteric coated encapsulated microspheres are:

- o Less inactivation of the preparation by acid and pepsin in the stomach
- o No need for simultaneous administration of antacids or H_2-receptor antagonists
- o More even distribution of the enzymes in chyme
- o More effective than conventional preparations
- o No hyperuricemia
- o Better patient compliance, probably because fewer tablets are required.

In spite of an increase in the lipase content, Eurobiol 25000 U®, like all other high-strength enzyme products, does not fully correct maldigestion and malabsorption. Possible causes of failure of normalization of lipid digestion are:

- o Delayed gastric emptying of the microspheres
- o Delay in the enzyme release from microspheres and even presence of intact enzyme microspheres in stool
- o Premature release of enzyme from microsphere in stomach.

One should remember that having optimal enzyme concentrations is not enough. These products should be bioavailable, and bioavailability depends upon several factors: source of enzyme (porcine, bovine, fungal), manufacturing process, stability, particle size of microspheres, gastric emptying time, intestinal pH and intestinal motility are other factors affecting bioavailability of enzyme preparations.

From this biophysiological background and a practical point of view we have to remember this new concept of duodenal bioavailability: microspheres should be gastric acid resistant to mechanical forces in stomach. The pH dependent opening of enteric coated preparation in the duodenum changes considerably the amount of product actually available in the site of action.

Clinical Results

The subsequent use of pancreatic supplement with a higher lipase content not only significantly reduces steatorrhea, but also creatorrhea. They have ipso facto a major impact on the nutritional status.

What are the facts about pancreatic enzymes?

- The "old-style" products are destroyed in stomach: only 15 to 22% of activity is found in the duodenum
- The classic Eurobiol® powder is more active: 30 to 56% of its activity is present in the distal half of the duodenum (Treitz corner)
- The enteric-coated preparations are more efficacious (+ 10% of fat absorption)
  It is easier to take them regularly (better compliance in children)
- The major activity of these new products is found not in the duodenum but in the ileum (maximum 4 hours after oral ingestion)
- The optimal dosage remains unknown.

We are also convinced that the concept "more is better" is erroneous, since the problem is not to reduce as far as possible the steatorrhea. The dose-response curve of pancreatic extracts is disappointing. Increasing the dosage provides little additional benefit but adds considerably to the cost of treatment, and perhaps also to toxic effects.

The commercial enzyme preparations available today are still not optimal. Their bioavailability depends on several factors that possibly change with the clinical condition from one patient to another.

Control of Efficacy

Most studies of pancreatic insufficiency have defined steator-rhea measured by Van de Kamer technique and documented clinically without enzyme supplement intake.

As pancreatic insufficiency progresses lipase activity in pancreas secretion diminishes at a faster rate than that of amylase or protease. In infants steatorrhea is defined by the following excretion of fat in the stool (without enzyme supplements):

- o >3.5 g/day   (children 0-18 months)
- o >5 g/day   (over 18 months)

Pancreatic enzyme replacement ist not only helpful in decreasing steatorrhea, but it is also used in the treatment of abdominal pain, discomfort and dyspepsia due to pancreatic disease and in the treatment of the distal intestinal obstruction syndrome (DIOS) complicating CF disease.

Improved nutrition, with an increase of body weight, indicates the positive effects of pancreatic enzymes. Many CF patients plan their own enzyme intake on the basis of subjective criteria, e.g. stool appearance and the presence of abdominal discomfort. Optimal absorption may be achieved with high-strength enteric-coated capsules, but we have to combine more frequent objective monitoring of nutritional status as reflected by the increase in body weight.

The great variability of the enzyme content and enzyme activity in commercial pancreatic supplements have also to be taken into consideration. As the manufacturers must ensure that their products contain a minimal dosage, stable for 6 months minimum, the variability is often positive, reaching up to 200% of the official dosage! This fact probably contributes to the "unexplained" clinical results in some studies.

Other factors that affect the bioavailability in vivo are interactions with other drugs and with food and between enzyme and co-enzyme. Thus regular measurement of activity in vivo does not reflect reality.

It is possible to measure:
- the weight of stool per day
- the steatorrhea
- the creatorrhea
- the percentage of fat absorption

It is also possible to measure the energy content of stool, nitrogen and fat absorption being calculated as the intake minus excretion expressed as percentage of intake. From the clinical point of view these calculations are rarely useful because they do not reflect reality. Normal pancreas, for example, secretes 600 000 units of lipase/day. This would be equivalent to more than 100 capsules/day of high-strength pancreatic extracts!

Better results are obtained from the comparison between fecal weight and stool energy loss rather than between fecal fat and stool energy loss. Two other pancreatic function tests may be useful: the measurement of the chymotrypsin level in stools and the PABA urine level after an oral PABA test.

Posology and the Rules of Prescription

In France only 3 preparations are available:

Products	Manu-facturer	Lipase	Protease	Amy-lase
Allpase *	Cilag	7500	600	5800
Créon *	Latema	12000	700	12000
Eurobiol 25000 U *	Jouveinal	25000	1250	22500

The majority of our colleagues have increased the dose for CF patients, but they do not prescribe more than 12 or 15 capsules per day of the high-strength preparation Eurobiol®, and perhaps it is appropriate not to exceed 250000 units per day. The important lesson of Dr. Smyth´s observations is that there is indeed an upper dose safety limit taking these high-strength pancreatic enzyme preparations, and that it is imperative to define this limit as well as to search for additional risk factors. ·

Children would probably need no more than 3 or 4 capsules per meal. We prefer to modify the diet intake, or find out why the pancreatic extracts do not work, rather than gradually increase the dosage.

In the UK many more preparations are available and the dosage given is much higher than in France. However, we believe this is not the sole factor in the recently described colonic strictures. Like all drugs, pancreatic enzyme preparations carry some risk.

We understand that in Canada, as in France, pancreatic enzyme preparations are prescribed according to the lipase content and the age of the patients.

Conclusion

- One of the goals of therapy is to ensure that optimal amounts of pancreatic enzyme supplements reach the duodenum.

- Care has to be taken to avoid too high a level of enzymes in the ileum. For this reason greater emphasis needs to be paid to routine assessment of total energy absorption rather than absorption of individual nutrients.

- We all need to work together in order to enhance the efficacy and decrease the risks of toxicity of the pancreatic enzyme enteric-coated preparations. The combined use of these enzymes with gastric acid resistant preparations and without may enhance efficacy. We further need a better knowledge of the bioavailability of these high-strength pancreatic enzymes, e.g., how different patients with CF react with regard to intestinal transit, hydration, bacterial overgrowth etc.

Table 2. Pancreatic enzyme preparations; proposed dosage according to the total lipase and the patient age

	Age	Preparation	Dosage
Infant	before 6 months	Eurobiol® powder	?
	6–18 months		2 000–4 000 U/meal
	(1 capsule/4 kg bodyweight of low preparation = Creon®)		
Children	1 to 6 years	between	4 000–6 000 or 8 000–12 000/meal
	after 7 years	basic:	4 000–8 000 or 8 000–12 000/meal
		plus	25 000 U in case of fat supplementation
daily		plus	6 000–12 000 U with Cyclo A 2x-3x daily

Table 3. Pancreatic enzyme preparations; official dosage according to the French Vidal-Book

	Preparation	Dosage
Adult with P.I.	Creon® 12 000 U :	4 to 8 capsules/day
	Eurobiol® 25 000:	(2), 4 to 6 capsules/day
(this is a base for CF)		

Children with CF receive more capsules, but never more than 12 to 15 capsules Eurobiol® 25 000.

Pathology of Colonic Cystic Fibrosis Obstructions

N. Brousse, J.C. Fournet, C. Silly, G. Lenoir, Paris

I have had the opportunity to go to Liverpool to see the slides of Dr. Smith's five cases representing strictures of ascending colon in cystic fibrosis. The lesions in all cases were remarkably similar. In fact, all were scarring lesions. The mucosa was nearly normal, and the most intriguing feature was the presence of an extensive fibrosis in the submucosa, which was the cause of the stenosis. Macroscopically, in one of these cases, the caecum was dilated, with widening of the submucosa.

Microscopically there were very few lesions in mucosa. Lesions in the submucosa were fibrous with little inflammation, and some areas of the muscular mucosa showed disruption. At higher magnification re-epithelialization of the surface epithelium could be seen. In some places one could see the muscular mucosa, this was the result of a previous ulceration going through the mucosa.

The pathogenesis of these strictures of the ascending colon were by no means clear. They could result from post-ischaemic ulceration repair initiated by pressure-induced dilation which in turn leads to mural ischaemia followed by ulceration and repair. The strictures may also be caused by an altered composition of the mucus, with a dehydrated abnormal lipid-free mucous mass. Is there direct local toxicity of the high-strength pancreatic enzymes? It is difficult to answer, because we have seen only healed lesions, with no or very little inflammation.

Looking at the literature on intestinal complications of cystic fibrosis, we found that many authors have described lesions either in the ileum or in the colon, resulting from partial or complete obstruction of the lumen by adherent material (inspissated intestinal secretions).

For nearly 30 years we have known that infants born with meconium ileus (5-15% of CF) are at increased risk of developing later distal intestinal obstruction. In fact half the cases of colonic strictures have been preceded by meconium ileus. It may be relevant that 25% of children and young adults with intestine complications of CF have meconium ileus equivalent. Faecaliths are fairly frequent in these children and young adult CF cases.

The late (i.e. post-neonatal) distal intestinal obstruction syndrome is characterized by abdominal pain due to constipation or faecal impaction. The obstructions by firm, putty-like faecal material which can completely block the bowel, are located in the terminal ileum and/or the right colon. They may be complicated by intussusception, even volvulus.

Chronic, recurrent small-intestinal obstruction occurs in about 20% of adult CF patients and has been variously ascribed to unusually large or fatty meal, accidental omission of pancreatin, by previous episodes of diarrhoea or dehydration.

Another author has described the meconium ileus equivalent in young children as occurring in the terminal ileum, the appendix and the caecum. In such cases no primary mucosal abnormality was described, but impacted faeces may be a cause.

Another complication of the distal intestinal obstruction syndrome is intussusception caused by a faecal bolus adherent to the mucosa. These lesions have been described only in the ileocaecal region.

Among our own records of CF we have found no cases of colonic stricture comparable to the Liverpool cases. However, we have reviewed three cases of intestinal obstruction syndrome in CF between 1970 and 1980, and I would like to give some details.

The first case is an 8-month-old boy who presented with an obstruction at the age of 4 months. 4 months later he suffered a second intestinal obstruction. This second intestinal obstruction appeared after the previous healed lesion, consisting of disruption of the muscular mucosa and fibrosis of the submucosa and the muscle layers. These lesions are due to previous ulceration (Fig. 1).

The second case is a 5-week-old girl who first presented with a neonatal occlusion leading to a perforation. 5 weeks later she presented with a second occlusion. At that time an ischaemic persistent lesion was seen in the mucosa associated with fibrosis of the submucosa and disruption of the muscular mucosa (Fig.2).

The last case is a 3-month-old boy who had atresia at birth. The segment above the atresia was narrowed and ischaemic.

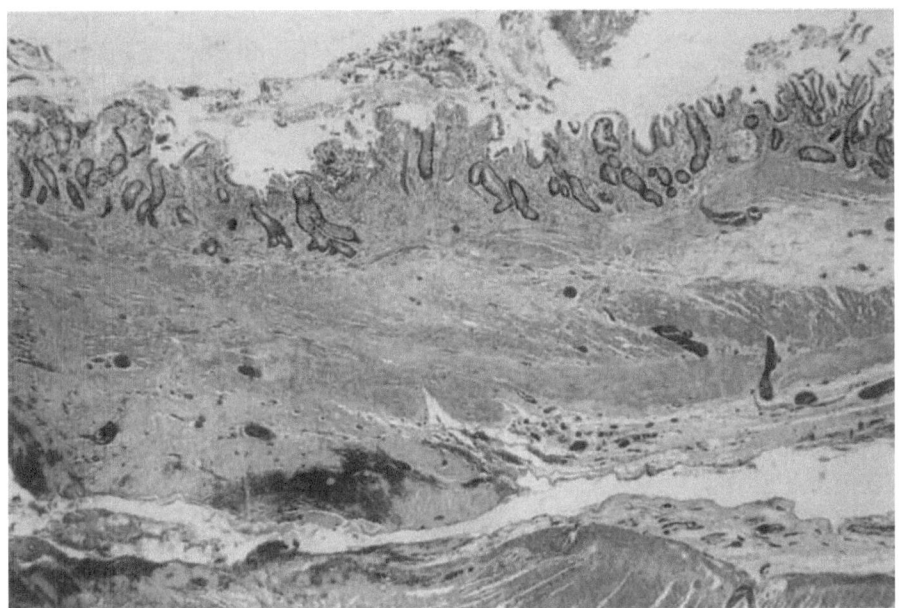

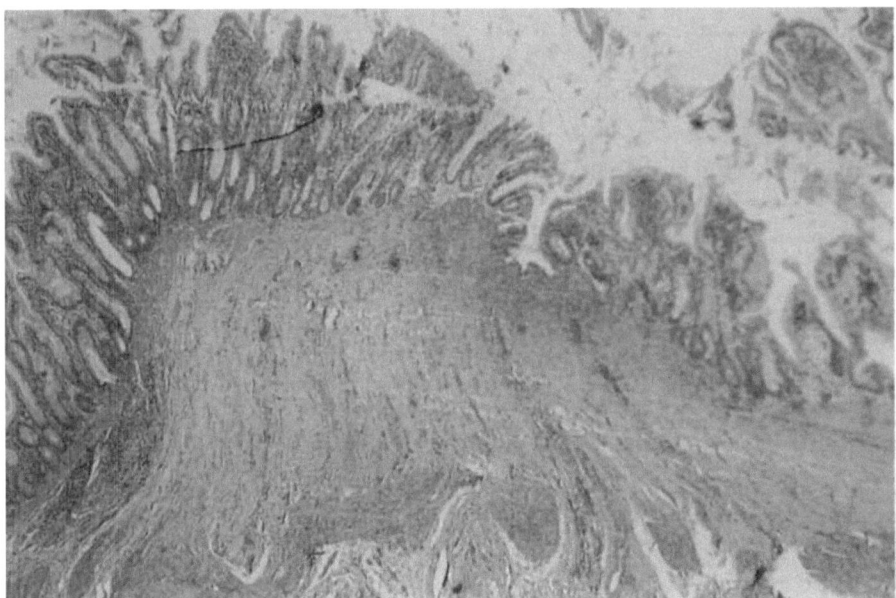

Fig. 1. Eight month-old-boy with cystic fibrosis: colonic obstruction occurring 4 months after a first colonic obstruction at the age of 4 months: the lesion, due to a previous ulceration, consists of disruption of the muscular mucosa and fibrosis of the submucosa

Fig. 2. Five week-old-girl with cystic fibrosis: colonic occlusion occurring 5 weeks after a first neo-natal occlusion: the lesion consists of an ischemic persistent lesion with disruption of the muscular mucosa and fibrosis of the submucosa

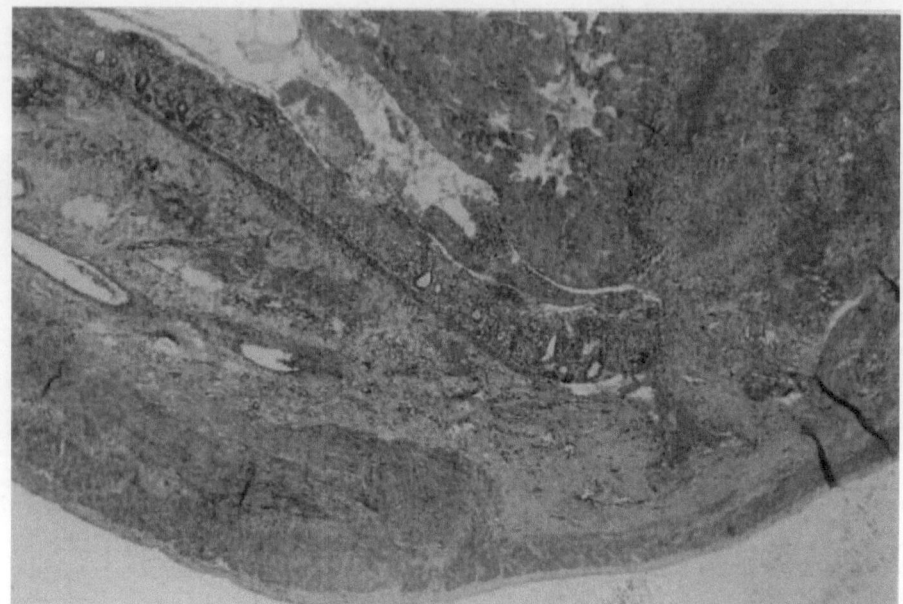

3

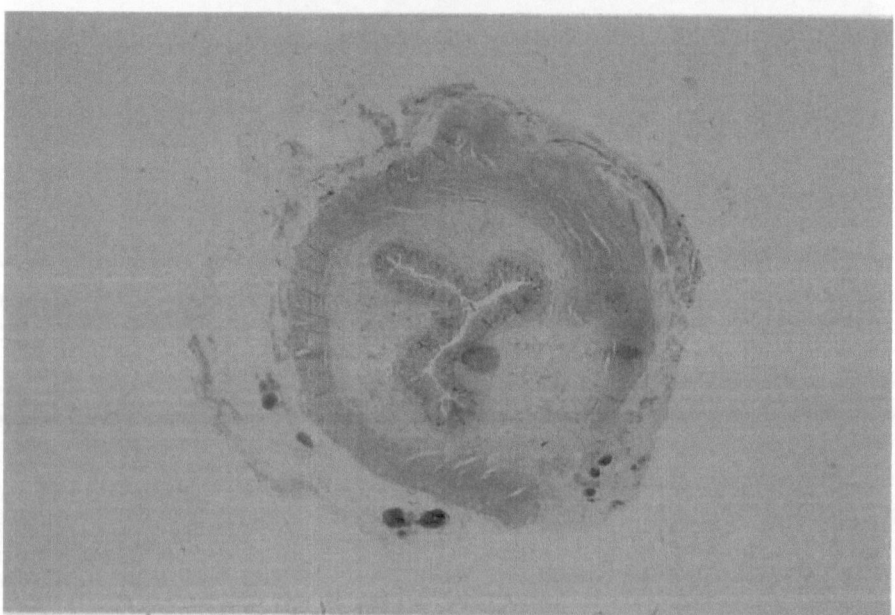

4

Fig. 3. Three month-old-boy with cystic fibrosis: intestinal atresia at birth. The segment above the atresia was narrowed. At autopsy, 3 months later, 2 colonic strictures were described: these stenoses were secondary to fibrous healed cicatrization of the previous mucosal ischemia. The lesion consists of mucosal ischemia, disruption of the muscular mucosa and fibrosis of the submucosa

Figs. 4–6. Young child without cystic fibrosis who presented repeated small intestinal and colonic strictures since birth, of unknown etiology. **Fig. 4** at low magnification, the lumen is very narrow; the submucosa is widening

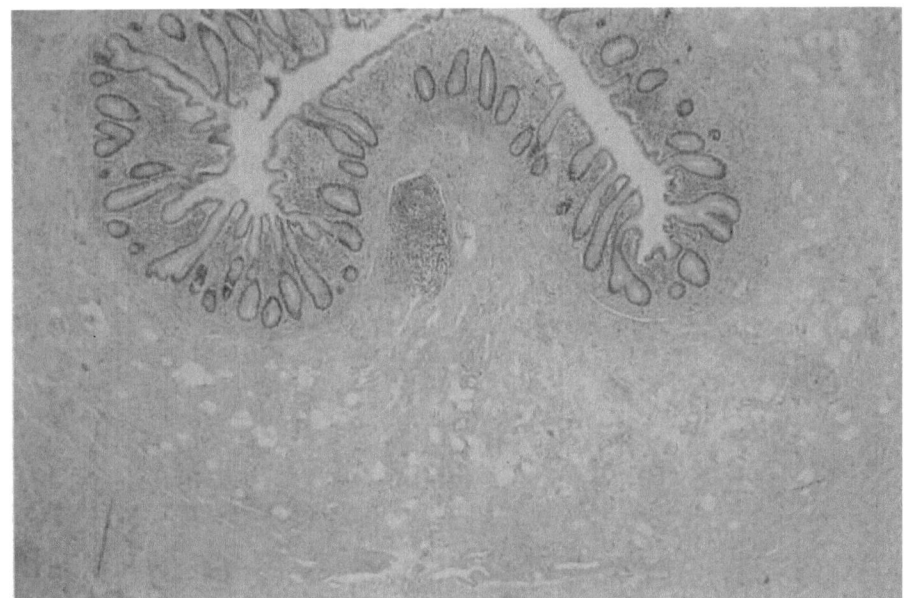

5

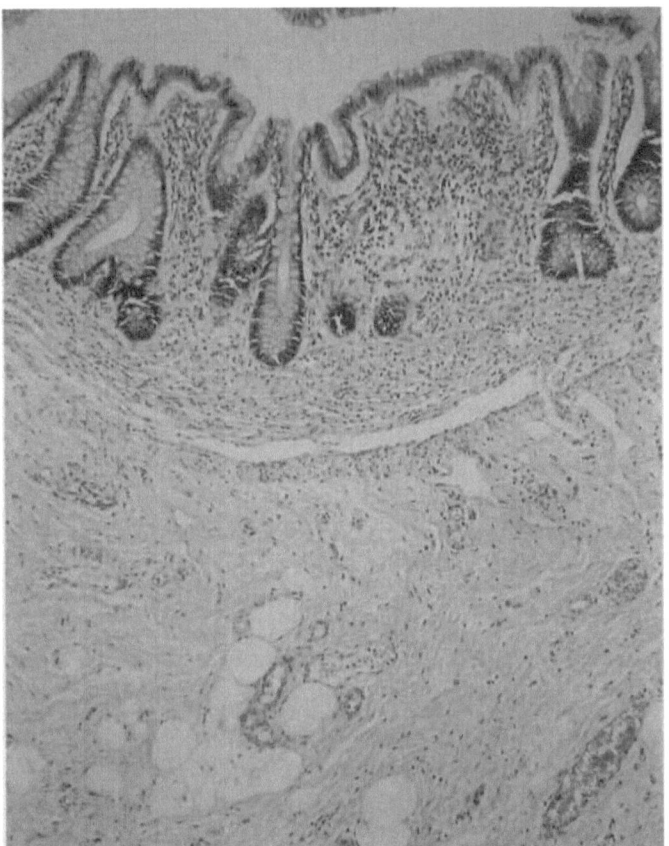

6

Fig. 5 at higher magnification, the mucosa is nearly normal, the submucosa is widening by fibrosis with very little information

Fig. 6 at higher magnification, the disruption of the muscular mucosa can be seen

3 months later he developed respiratory failure and died. At autopsy two colonic stenoses with stricture were described. These stenosis were secondary to fibrous healed cicatriation of the previous mucosal ischaemia (Fig. 3).

I also want to present the case of a child without cystic fibrosis who has had two repeated small intestinal and colonic strictures since birth. We do not know the aetiology of these strictures. The histological picture of the colonic stricture is exactly the same as that described in the Liverpool cases - namely, scarring lesions with submucosa fibrosis. This young child without cystic fibrosis presented at age 9 months with the same symptoms and signs, stenosis of the lumen, with widening of the submucosa and a normal mucosa. At a higher magnification the mucosa is nearly normal, but there is disruption of the muscular mucosa and fibrosis of the submucosa. There is a little inflammation with a few polymorphs and some eosinophils (Figs. 4–6).

So, in the cases we have seen the histology was identical with that of the submucosal scarring lesions seen in the Liverpool series. The cause could be either CF mechanical obstruction in the ileocaecal region, leading to ulcerations, secondary intussusception and healing, or it could be a direct chemical effect related to enzyme toxicity. Since we did not see any inflammation but only healed lesions, I think it would be better to do a prospective study of CF cases looking for intestinal pathology.

Prof. Dodge: The case of the child without cystic fibrosis is fascinating. Has anyone inquired whether the parents have been giving this baby pancreatic enzymes for any reason?

Prof. Brousse: He has been in the hospital since birth.

Prof. Dodge: Well, I admit it is unlikely, but we have had children in hospital who have been poisoned by their parents with drugs without anyone knowing. I think it is unlikely, but it just needs to be excluded because if it can be excluded then we are into a very interesting area of aetiology.

Prof. Brousse: I cannot answer your question precisely. The only question I asked the clinician was "Is there any cystic fibrosis?", and the answer was "No". I did not ask about the enzymes.

One Year Monitoring of a Lipase Rich Pancreatic Enzyme Preparation (Enzipan®) in the Treatment of Severe Lipid Maldigestion of Cystic Fibrosis

M. Antonelli, S. Bertasi, M. Matrunola, P. Canuzzi, Rome

Pancreatic insufficiency is a cardinal feature of cystic fibrosis (CF), and 90% of CF patients require pancreatic enzyme supplementation, with a wide interpatient variation in the dosage. Many patients consume large quantities of enzyme capsules in order to prevent steatorrhoea, reduce the number and bulk of stools and improve nutrition and growth [1].

Enteric coated microsphere (ECM) preparations have become the treatment of choice of CF maldigestion [2], but large numbers of capsules may be required to reduce faecal loss, and this often leads to poor compliance [3].

In spite of large doses of enzyme supplements in several CF patients, dietary lipid absorption and weight gain may remain unsatisfactory and abdominal pain unrelieved. It is thus suggested that the advent of high-lipase enzymes may offer the advantages of a smaller number of capsules, better nutrition and improved compliance.

We studied the efficacy and tolerability of a new lipase-rich enteric coated (ECMT) preparation (Enzipan®)* (containing 25 000 units (U.F. EUR) of lipase activity per capsule) in CF patients with severe steatorrhoea, who had not achieved a lipid absorption coefficient (LAC) of 90% with an ECM formulation containing 5000 units of lipase activity, for a period of 12 months.

Patients and Methods

Twelve outpatients (8 male, 4 female) attending the CF centre were enrolled in the study. The age range was 11 to 25 years

---

* Provided by Ravizza Farmaceutici Spa, Italy.

(mean 16.4 years). All patients had symptoms of CF and at least two sweat chloride concentrations > 60 mmol (mEq/l) LAC < 90% and severe steatorrhoea (mean 23.6 g fat/day at baseline) inadequately reduced (to the target of 19 g/day), in spite of a personally adjusted full-dose pancreatic supplementation with an ECM preparation during meals. Patients with severe disease rendering normal enteral feeding impossible, or associated complications (liver cirrhosis, diabetes, increased abdominal pain) affecting the efficacy of treatment, were excluded. Verbal informed consent was obtained from all patients and/or their parents.

Treatment Schedule

At the time of enrolment patients were on an unrestricted fat-rich diet (mean 39 + 5 Kcal %) and individual ECM therapy, at a mean of 23 capsules per day and with a lipase mean daily content of 113 300 + 16 143 units.

Each patient was given Enzipan® at a mean dose of 12 capsules (half the number of ECM capsules), corresponding to a mean daily lipase intake of 302 083 + 71 078 units for 12 consecutive months. Each Enzipan® capsule contains 25 000 units (FIP) of lipase activity, 22 500 units of amylase activity and 1250 units of proteolytic activity.

Methods of Assessment

Efficacy of ECMT was evaluated every 2 months by measurement of:

- body weight
- body mass percentile (BMP)

and half yearly evaluation of:

- LAC
- steatorrhoea
- height

A constant fat-rich diet was maintained during the study period. The diet and its lipid content were recorded daily on a dietary chart and were assessed every 3 months. Stools for steatorrhoea (3-day faecal collection) and LAC analysis were collected before the start of treatment, after 6 months and at the end of study. Stool fat was determined by the method of Van de Kamer [4].

LAC was calculated according to the following formula:

$$\frac{\text{Fat intake (g) - Fat excretion}}{\text{Fat intake (g)}} \times 100\%$$

Values were reported as percent absorption (coefficient of fat absorption x 100). Concomitant medication with antisecretory agents and antacids was not permitted; antibiotics, vitamins and other treatments for CF were maintained throughout the study period. Abdominal ultrasound examinations were performed every 2 months and whenever meconium ileus equivalent symptoms (colicky abdominal pain, a right lower quadrant mass) and/or signs of intestinal obstruction occurred.

Tolerability and Safety

These were evaluated on the basis of patients' complaints or a change in intestinal symptoms such as flatus, abdominal pain, abdominal distension or bowel movements. Clinical acceptability was assessed by recorded daily dosage of medication and evaluated by the investigators.

Blood urea nitrogen, blood urea, creatinine, plasma, uric acid concentrations and liver function tests were done every two months.

Statistical Analysis

The pre-treatment comparability of Enzipan®, changes in LAC and changes in non-digested and non-absorbed fat, lipase units x gram of ingested fat x day, body mass index and % ideal weight x height were analysed with the Wilcoxon rank test.

The variations in number of capsules and lipase units ingested per day were analysed with Student's t test; variations in uricaemia were analysed with the Mann-Whitney test.

Results

During the study all patients were maintained on a hypercaloric fat-rich (40 + 1.1 Kcal %) diet. The mean starting daily dosage of Enzipan® of 12 capsules was reduced to 10 during the first 2 months of therapy, resulting in very significant decrease ($p<0.0001$) in the mean number of capsules taken daily, compared with the 23 ECM capsules previously taken.

Table 1. Comparative values of lipase units per day, lipase units per gram of ingested fat, of absorbed fats and nondigested fats number of capsules

	Lipase* (mean ± sem)		Fats % absorbed (means ± sem)	Faecal fats g/day (mean ± sem)	(mean ± sem)
	U/FIP	U/gr Fats			
Standard	113.3 ± 4.6	1.17 ± 0.11	23 ± 0.9	80.8 ± 8	19 ± 9.5
Lipase rich					
Starting	302 ± 20.5	2.67 ± 0.3	12 ± 0.8	90.7 ± 3.7	10.7 ± 4.7
Assessed	264 ± 24.8	2.12 ± 0.2	10.5 ± 0.9		

* U/FIP and U/g Fats x 1000

The total mean daily lipase activity load (U/FIP) presented a threefold increase, from 113 000 units per day, when on ECM, to 302 000 units per day (p<0.0001) at the beginning of Enzipan® administration. The dose was then reduced to a mean of 214 000 units per day because of abdominal complaints in some patients, and the difference was significant (p<0.0001). The lipase activity units/g of daily ingested fat increased from a mean of 1170 units when taking ECM to 2120 units (p=0.002) when patients switched to an adjusted dose of Enzipan® supplementation. Mean faecal fat loss fell significantly from 19 g/24 h in the pre-treatment period to 10 g/24 h

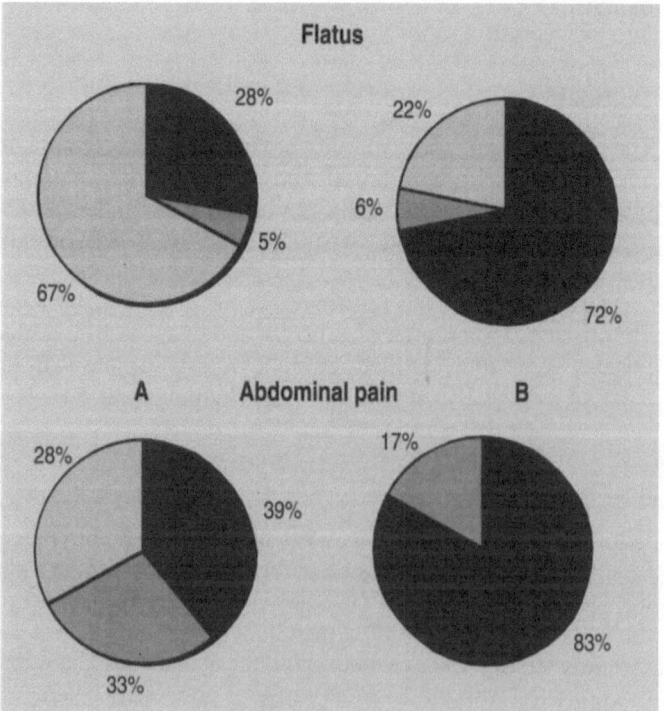

Fig. 1. Variations in flatus and abdominal pain observed in the pretreatment period (**A**) versus lipase rich preparation (**B**).
moderate
slight ■
absent ■

Flatus

28% 22%
5% 6%
67% 72%

A Abdominal pain B

28% 17%
39%
33% 83%

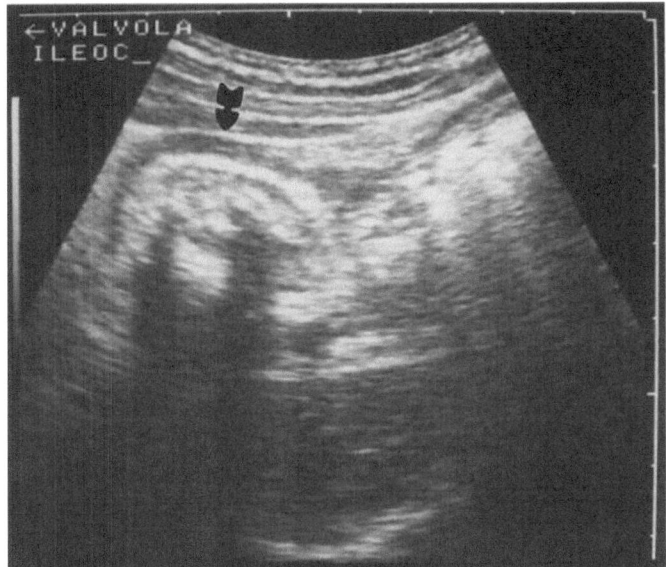

Fig. 2. Oedema with thickening of caecum wall and faecal impaction in a CF patient receiving more than 2 200 lipase units per gram of ingested fat

(p=0.006). Mean LAC rose significantly from the baseline value of 80% to 90% (p=0.006) (Table 1).

There were no abnormalities in laboratory findings except for mean blood urea concentrations, which progressively rose from a baseline value of 4.6 g/dl to 5.8 g/dl after 6 months and to 6.6 g/dl after 1 year (p=0.01); however, they remained within the normal range. The influence of Enzipan® on body weight was evaluated by dividing patients into two subgroups, those under 18 years (n=7) and those over 19 years (n=5). In the first group weight gain was evaluated according to the % of ideal weight x height formula, and a non-significant statistical increase of this index, from 81 to 87 (p=0.068), was observed. In the latter group the body mass index, the most appropriate for this age, showed a statistically non-significant increase (p=0.18) from a baseline value of 19.4 to 20.4 after 1 year of treatment.

Enzipan® was more acceptable to all patients than ECM. Seven patients expressed concern about offensive stools and abdominal pain in the first 2 months of the study.

The reduction of the dose of Enzipan® relieved the abdominal symptoms and restored normal bowel function. Patients' daily diaries showed a marked reduction of self-perceived abdominal symptoms, e.g. 95% reported flatus in the pre-treatment period, falling to 28% while on Enzipan®; 61% had abdominal pain, often disturbing, before treatment, compared with 17% during treatment (Fig.1).

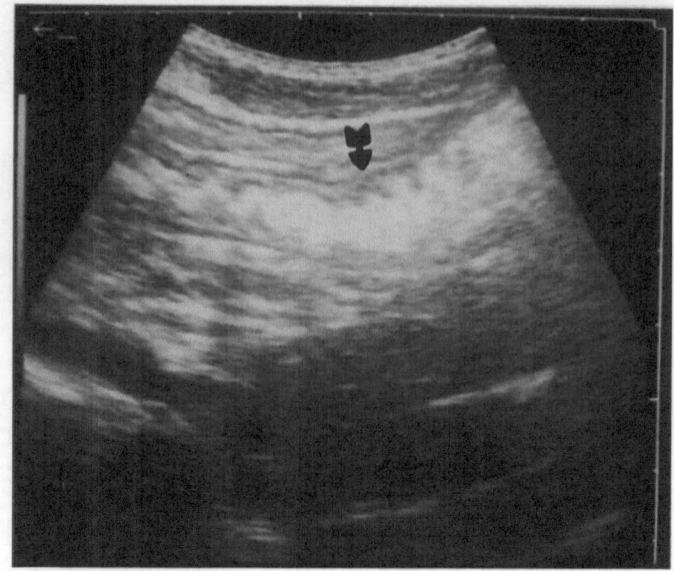

Fig. 3. CF patient receiving more than 2 200 lipase units per gram of ingested fat. Oedema and thickening wall of transverse colon with marked austrae. The lumen is filled with faeces

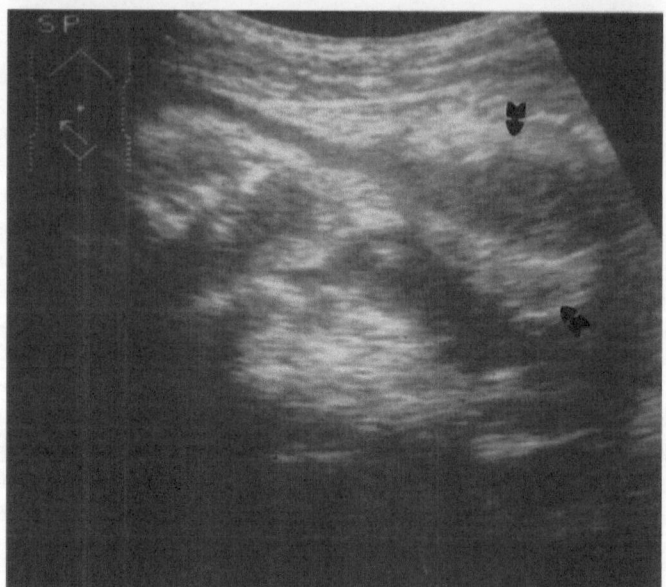

Fig. 4. Marked thickening of caecum and appendix abscess

Abdominal ultrasound examination every 2 months revealed at various times throughout the study unexpected and symptomless thickening of the distal intestinal wall in four patients (Fig.2), associated with thickening of the ascending-transverse colonic wall in three (Fig.3). All were on individually tailored doses of Enzipan®, containing lipase activity/g of daily ingested fat higher than 2 200 units. Three had previously experienced symptoms of distal intestinal obstruction [5]. In the past, all these patients had irregular eating habits, character-

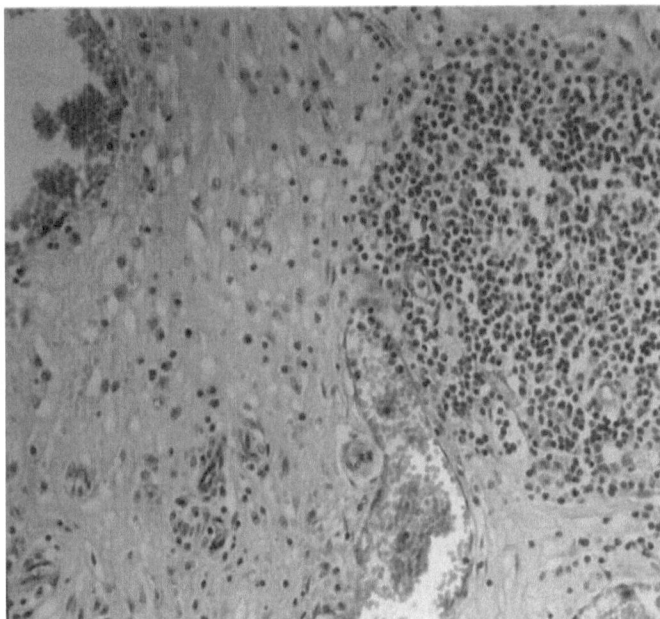

Fig. 5. Microscopic pattern of acute inflammation and abscess in the appendix wall (x 10000)

ized by ingestion of prescribed doses of enzymes at each mealtime even when the meal was reduced in quantity or omitted. The reduction of lipase dose below 2000 units/g of ingested fat and closer supervision of the food intake within 2 weeks led to complete restoration of the normal features of the ileal and colonic walls. One patient during the 11th month of Enzipan® therapy presented a painful mass in the right lower quadrant of the abdomen and reduced appetite. An ultrasound abdominal examination showed progressive thickening of the terminal portion of ileum and an appendix abscess (Fig.4). The patient underwent surgery and the diagnosis of appendicitis and typhlitis was confirmed (Fig.5).

Discussion

Short-term studies of the efficacy of lipase rich pancreatic preparations [6,7] have shown that these formulations are superior to the previous standard lipase potency (5000 units) preparations in reducing faecal fat excretion and in improving LAC. The advantage is the marked reduction in dosage, which is likely to improve patients' convenience, compliance and life style, especially of those obliged to take large amounts of medication each day. No information about the efficacy in relieving subjective complaints, such as frequency and intensity of abdominal pain and flatus, was given in these studies.

The present study shows that the long-term use of the lipase-rich preparation Enzipan® in CF patients presenting high residual fat loss was effective in decreasing non-digested fat levels and in improving LAC and to a lesser extent nutrition in CF patients when compared with values previously obtained with a conventional ECM preparation. Of particular importance are the significant reductions in faecal fat loss (p=0.006) and the increase in LAC to normal values (p=0.06). This confirms that in many CF patients there is a portion of fat malabsorption that is not controlled even by large doses of ECM preparations. There was also a marked reduction in flatus and abdominal pain, which could promote a better body image and life style.

Conventional criteria for calculating the dose of pancreatic supplements is at present based on daily lipase needs [7] or on the fat content of an average adult meal [1]. The experience gained with prolonged use of Enzipan® demonstrates the inadequacy of these criteria. A more reliable criterion based on fat intake with diet and its distribution with meals is needed, as is a more careful and constant monitoring of patients' diet to promote a fat rich diet. In particular, it is advisable to identify how many lipase units are required for optimal digestion of 1 g of ingested fat so that the total dose of enzymes, and how it should be apportioned between individual meals, can be established and side effects or intestinal complications more easily avoided.

Recently eight CF patients (seven from England and one from Denmark) have been reported to have a fibrotic stricture of ascending colon [8,9], after 12-15 months of lipase high strength enzyme preparations. Seven of these required surgery. Since this report there has been growing concern about the safety of these preparations.

The present study demonstrates that the optimal lipase dose ranges between 1500 and 2000 units/g of lipid intake, and with this dosage no signs or symptoms of intestinal obstruction were observed. Thus it may be deduced that those patients who presented colonic narrowing, corresponding to scarring of the large intestine [8], had consumed an uncontrolled "hyperdosage" of lipase-rich enzyme. This criterion was also useful for adjusting the dose of enzymes to the amount of fat taken with each meal and was indirectly valuable in identifying overdosage in the symptom-free phase in four patients.

Abdominal ultrasound examinations every 2 months showed a thickening of the wall of the terminal portion of the ileum in four patients, associated with the same finding in the ascending and transverse colon in three. No luminal stricture was demonstrated. The strictures disappeared after Enzipan® was reduced below 2000 units/g of ingested fat. The reduction of lipase dosage was decided on the basis of food intake and its lipid content, revealing in each patient the ingestion, in most meals, of a lipase load of 2300-2700 units/g of dietary fat for at least 1 month. The potential adverse effect of excessive and repeated doses of enzymes on the colonic wall could otherwise be explained by the observation that in patients with pancreatic insufficiency the ingested lipase is caudally displaced [10]. Thus the enzyme activity is inappropriately low in the duodenum and too high in the ileum so that unutilized but already active lipase wasting into the colon becomes inevitable.

Current concern about the safety of these preparations requires further study to elucidate the mechanism underlying the narrowing of the colon, and to identify preventive measures. In order to extrapolate from the results of our study an appropriate measure for rational dosage and for easier prevention of side effects, including colonic stricture, during enzyme-rich formulation consumption, we suggest:

A) Careful selection of patients. The most suitable candidates for lipase-rich preparations are those who need more than 5 capsules of ECM at each meal, who present LAC < 90 and have high residual fat loss (> 10 g/day).
B) Careful dietary advice with a recommendation of a lipid-rich diet, and accurate recording of daily food intake.
C) Frequent three-day diet recalls.
D) Correlation of the number of lipase units to the quantity of fat ingested at each meal.
E) Constant and regular count of capsules ingested with each meal.
F) Ultrasound examination of the abdomen every 2 months, or earlier if symptoms of distal intestinal obstruction syndrome (DIOS) appear.
G) An average dosage of 1000 lipase units/g of fat. (Individual response should be judged by signs and symptoms (appetite, bowel movements, reduction of abdominal symptoms) and objective parameters (e.g. nutrition, stools, steatorrhoea, abdominal scanning.)
H) Maximum dose should not exceed 2000 lipase units/g of ingested fat and should be adjusted on the basis of clinical control and constant monitoring of dietary composition and intake per meal, with the support of programmed abdominal ultrasound examinations.

References

1. George DE, Mangos JA (1988) Nutritional management and pancreatic Enzyme Therapy in Cystic Fibrosis: State of the art in 1987 and Projections into the Future. J of Pediat Gastroenter and Nutr (Suppl 1): S 49–57
2. Beverley DW, Kelleher J, Macdonald A, Littlewood JM, Robinson T, Walters MP (1987) Comparison of four pancreatic extracts in cystic fibrosis. Arch Dis Child: 62, 564–568
3. Brady MS, Rickard K, Yup L, Eigen H (1991) Effectiveness and safety of small vs large doses of enteric coated pancreatic enzymes in reducing steatorrhoea in children with Cystic Fibrosis: a prospective randomized study. Pediatric Pulmonology: 10, 79–85
4. Van de Kamer JM, Huinink HTB, Weyers HA (1949) Rapid method for the determination of fat in feces. J Biol Chem: 117, 347–355
5. Mathese JW, Go VLW, Di Magno EP (1977) Meconium ileus equivalent. Complicating in postneonatal children and young adults: report of 12 cases. Gastroenterology: 72, 732–736
6. Shah A, Diiuwiddie R, Madges S, Prescott P, Hudsong (1993) High dose Nutrizym 22 in Cystic fibrosis. Eur J Pediatr: 152, 763–764
7. Chazalette JP (1993) A double blind placebo controlled trial of a pancreas Enzyme formulation (Panzytrat® 25 000) in the treatment of impaired lipid digestion in patients with Cystic Fibrosis. Drug Invest: 5 (5), 274–280
8. Smith RL, Van Velzen D, Smith AR, Lloid DL, Heaf DP (1994) Strictures of ascending colon in cystic fibrosis and high strength pancreatic enzymes. Lancet: 343, 85–86
9. Committee on Safety of medicines (1993) Personal communication
10. Guarner L, Rodriguez R, Guarner F, Malagelada JR (1993) Fate or oral enzymes in pancratic insufficiency. GUT: 34, 708–712

J. M. Littlewood, St. James, Leeds

1. The following factors are considered when determining the dose of pancreatic enzymes (Littlewood, 1994):

   - age, body weight and weight for height of the child.
   - the adequacy and previous rate of growth.
   - dietary energy and constituents, particularly the fat intake.
   - clinical evidence of malabsorption e.g. abdominal symptoms of pain, intolerance of fatty foods, character of stools, abdominal distension and nutritional state.
   - laboratory evidence of malabsorption e.g. fat microscopy for neutral and split fat (Walters et al, 1990), quantitative faecal fat measurements (Gilbert et al, 1988), faecal chymotrypsin values. These measurements are repeated as the dose of enzymes is gradually increased.
   - the contribution that the chest infection may be making to the energy needs.

   The patients are mostly without symptoms, are absorbing 85 to 90% of ingested fat and are in a good nutritional state (around mean for age) (Littlewood and Wolfe, 1994).

2. The units of lipase required by the average patient are taken into consideration although there is great variation between patients. The amount of enzyme per meal will vary for the individual patient as they are encouraged to take more enzymes with a fatty meal or snack.

   It is helpful to consider units of lipase/kg body weight/day and the units of lipase/gm of fat ingested as these can identify patients taking excessive doses.

3. The amount of fat taken by the patient is rarely, if ever, limited these days. Patients are encouraged to take as much fat as they can manage. As this is contrary to the present day advice for a "healthy diet", they are reassured that fat malabsorption is never completely corrected and that the amount of fat absorbed is not enough to increase their chances of developing arterial disease.

High fat diets (fat supplying more than 40% of the total energy intake) are rarely achieved. Derestriction of dietary fat intake merely achieves a normal fat intake. Our clinic patients derive 37% of energy from fat, on average.

4. Enzymes are given in capsules, half at the start and half in the middle of the meal. This is standard practice in our clinic and is followed by all patients (Brady et al, 1992).

   For infants the enzymes are taken out of their capsules and given as a bolus in a little liquid, fruit puree or a small amount of soft food at the start of the meal or feed - NOT sprinkled on or mixed with all the food or the whole formula feed. Young children are encouraged to take the enzymes in the capsule; many are able to swallow the capsules by the age of 5 years. Enzymes should, of course, be also taken with snacks.

5. Enzymes do not seem to interact with other medications, although diarrhoea from a course of antibiotics may interfere with adjustment of enzyme dose. Intravenous antibiotics in particular may affect the bowels. However, this is not a practical difficulty. The only other important relationship of enzymes to oral drugs has been the need for transplant patients to take enzymes with their cyclosporin.

6. The effectiveness of enzyme replacement therapy is judged first by the control of abdominal symptoms and signs, e.g. pain, distension, stool character and frequency. In our clinic only a minority of children (approximately 10%) taking enzymes have gastrointestinal pain, distention or abnormal stools; their symptoms are usually mild and infrequent.

   More objective assessment involves faecal microscopy for neutral and split fat and chymotrypsin estimation. When the chymotrypsin is normal (>120 μg/gm) and the neutral fat has cleared, a formal faecal fat collection is made at the same time as a dietary assessment, to allow calculation of the percentage absorption of ingested fat. Usually between 85% and over 90% fat absorption is achieved with optimal doses of enzymes. Faecal fats are estimated annually as part of the "birthday assessment". Periodic faecal fat microscopy and chymotrypsins are checked at clinic visits if there are gastrointestinal symptoms or suboptimal weight gain or nutritional state. Detailed enquiries about the gastrointestinal tract and abdominal examination are made at every clinic visit.

7. The marked faecal fat estimations are accurate and helpful (Gilbert et al, 1988). Faecal fat microscopy, described above,

has also been well validated in our unit (Walters et al, 1990) and is a cheap and most helpful investigation. We are surprised that many of our colleagues do not use this semi-quantitative method of monitoring fat absorption - particularly for adult patients who are reluctant to do standard faecal collections. Many patients have suboptimally controlled absorption on referral to our unit because there has been no attempt to monitor their faecal fat output (Littlewood, 1993). Subjective assessments give a more crude indication of absorption and frequently fail to identify even severe malabsorption.

8. Compliance is variable with all forms of treatment. We suspect that compliance with enzymes is good in most patients because they develop unpleasant symptoms if the enzymes are omitted. Our main experience with poor compliance is in young children who may go through "enzyme refusal stages". There may also be problems with school age children who need to take large doses of enzymes in front of their peers. Experience with adults suggests that enzyme compliance is good, in contrast to nebuliser treatment and physiotherapy. Chronic compliance problems are not a major cause of poor control of malabsorption in children with cystic fibrosis.

9. Our patients are advised to take a high energy diet with liberal quantities of fat and protein.

Age (yrs)	(n)	Percent ($\pm$ SD) estimated average energy requirement
0– 5	21	119 (35)
6–10	34	128 (24)
11–15	41	130 (27)

Nutritional intake of patients attending St James

To achieve a good nutritional state it is still necessary for patients to take a higher than normal energy intake, even with the better enzymes and more aggressive treatments for respiratory infections now available (Wolfe et al, 1994). The traditional advice to take between 120 and 150% of the normally recommended energy intake for age are still appropriate but should of course be tailored to individual requirements.

Nutritional supplements may be required to achieve these high energy intakes, which are necessary for normal growth and nutritional state; in our clinic 68% of patients

Age	(n)	%Wt/Ht	%Wt/Age	%Ht/Age	Wt SD	Ht SD
0-5	21	96.1	101.0	102.7	+0.1	+0.8
6-10	34	100.9	101.3	99.1	+0.1	+0.1
11-15	41	98.6	95.6	98.0	-0.2	-0.4

take such supplements. Early consideration is given to nasogastric or gastrostomy feeding if weight gain is poor.

10. In our clinic the methods of diagnosis used were as follows: gastrointestinal malabsorption (44% of patients), respiratory infections (23%), meconium ileus (14%), neonatal screening (13%), sibling affected (13%).

   The mode of presentation seems to influence the frequency of abdominal symptoms in patients who are referred to our unit for comprehensive assessment (Littlewood, 1993).

11. All patients have their genotype characterised, and the vast majority in the North of England are homozygous (75%) or heterozygous (22%) for ΔF508. Although certain mild mutations are more likely to be associated with pancreatic "sufficiency", this knowledge has no practical use in the individual patient at the present time.

12. Meconium ileus was the presenting feature in 14% of our clinic patients. So called "meconium ileus equivalent" or distal intestinal obstruction syndrome is rarely seen in patients attending the clinic, where only a minority of children have any gastrointestinal symptoms on either standard or high lipase enzyme preparations. Abdominal pain is commonly related to constipation if the absorption is corrected, the patients developing a variety of acquired megacolon (Littlewood, 1992).

13. During recent years the growth and development of our CF children has been virtually normal (see above). The nutritional state of patients referred from elsewhere has also improved, but to a lesser extent (Littlewood, 1993). The growth and development of CF infants diagnosed following neonatal screening in our hospital has been normal(Simmonds et al, 1993).

14. When colonic complications of high lipase preparations are suspected we use ultrasound, gastrografin follow-through, barium enema and colonoscopy. The gastrografin follow-through has proved a useful alternative to barium enema and is less unpleasant for the patient. The

investigation consists of serial abdominal X-rays after oral gastrografin; often the colon is clearly outlined in later films, sparing the child a barium enema. Our radiologist is less impressed with the value of ultrasound than suggested in the Liverpool report.

Since early in 1994, when most of our children were taking high lipase preparations, any who had any abnormal gastrointestinal symptoms have been investigated as follows:

* faecal fat microscopy
* faecal chymotrypsin
* faecal occult blood
* abdominal ultrasound
* gastrografin follow-through
* barium enema (if colon not visualised with gastrografin)

15. Two children with colonic strictures presented with chronic abdominal symptoms, one with pain the other with pain and abnormal stools (Green et al, 1994, Archives of Disease in Childhood, in press).

Case 1

A 5-year-old boy had meconium ileus for which two segments of ileum (3.8 cm and 5.5 cm) were resected on the second day and an ileostomy made. A further 25 cm of ileum, including the ileocaecal valve, were resected at 5 weeks. He was referred to our clinic at 3 yr 4 m when he had persistent very offensive diarrhoea, poor appetite and deteriorating chest disease. A barium enema was normal. He was treated first with Creon 25 000, 25 capsules/day, and then with Pancrease HL, 20-28 capsules/day. His stools remained very loose and offensive. He gained little weight over the next year and at times he was taking up to 40 Pancrease HL/day (66 000 lipase/kg/day and 3300 units protease/kg/day).

At 4 yr 8 m he passed some blood in the stool. He was changed at standard Creon, 35 capsules/day. A repeat barium enema demonstrated an extensive stricture from the remaining ascending colon to the lower descending colon. Ultrasound demonstrated thickening of the bowel wall of the transverse and descending colon.

At laparotomy the colon appeared thickened. An ileostomy was formed and full thickness biopsies were taken. Biopsies showed mild subserosal fibrosis and very prominent deep submucosal fibrosis. The mucosa showed a mild diffuse colitis. On enteral nutrition his abdominal pain has ceased, but there is still a large output from his ileostomy; the colon will be inspected again after six months.

Case 2

A girl aged 7 yr 2 m was diagnosed at 2 yr 4 m, presenting with diarrhoea, poor weight gain and chronic cough. She was referred with a chronic collapse of the right middle lobe, which was eventually removed. She had intermittent abdominal pain despite adequate control of the malabsorption. Gradual increase in dose and changes in enzyme preparation ended with a dose of Pancrease HL 27 capsules/day at 7 years.

At this time a barium enema revealed moderate narrowing and lack of distensibility of the ascending colon, but ultrasound was normal. At colonoscopy the mucosa in the ascending colon was slightly reddened, but histology was normal, as was that of the terminal ileum. She reverted to standard Pancrease (27/day) and is well, her pain having improved.

16. There are insufficient patients with abdominal symptoms to suggest seasonal variation.

17. There has been no case of Crohn's disease in 500 patients with CF assessed at our clinic.

18. All patients are on long term flucloxacillin as anti-staphylococcal prophylaxis. For "colds", patients who do not have *Pseudomonas aeruginosa* have amoxycillin or a similar antibiotic added, depending on the organism and sensitivity; those who are infected with *P. aeruginosa* usually have a course of ciprofloxacin. Exacerbations of chest infection are treated with intravenous antibiotics - either tobramycin with azlocillin or ceftazidime or two antibiotics appropriate to the bacterial sensitivities. Half the patients receive long-term nebulised antibiotics twice daily.

19. Histology of the two patients who had colonic strictures is available (Green et al, 1994).

References

1. Brady MS, Richard K, Yu P, Eigen (1992) Effectiveness of enteric coated pancreatic enzyme supplements given before meals in reducing steatorrhoea in children with cystic fibrosis. J Am Diet Assoc 1992;92:813-817

2. Gilbert J, Kelleher J, Walters MP, Littlewood JM. Markers for faecal fat estimation in monitoring steatorrhoea in cystic fibrosis. Gut 188; 29:1286-1288

3. Green MR, Southern KW, Wolfe SP, Smith SEW, Najmaldin AZ, Wyatt JI, Littlewood JM (1994) Colonic strictures in children with cystic fibrosis. Submitted for publication to Arch Dis Child 1994

4. Littlewood JM (1991) Pancreatic enzymes in cystic fibrosis. In: Lankisch PG (ED): Pancreatic Enzymes in Health and Disease. Springer, Berlin, Heidelberg, 1991;177-187

5. Littlewood JM (1992) Gastrointestinal complications in cystic fibrosis. J Roy Soc Med 1992;85(suppl 18):13-19

6. Littlewood JM (1993) Value of comprehensive assessment and investigation in cystic fibrosis. In: Escobar H, Baquero F, Suarez L (eds). Clinical Ecology of Cystic Fibrosis. Elsevier Science Pub. B.V. 1993;181-187

7. Littlewood JM, Wolfe SP (1994) Nutrition in cystic fibrosis. In: Heatley RV, Green JH, Losowsky MS (eds). Consensus in Clinical Nutrition. Churchill Livingstone, 1994

8. Smyth RL, van Velzen D, Smyth AR, Lloyd DA, Heaf DP (1994) Strictures of ascending colon in cystic fibrosis and high-strength pancreatic enzymes. Lancet 1994;343:85-86

9. Walters MP, Kelleher J, Gilbert J, Littlewood JM (1990) Clinical monitoring of steatorrhoea in cystic fibrosis. Arch Dis Child 1990;65:99-102

10. Wolfe SP. Unpublished data, 1994.

Chicago Experience of Intestinal Strictures and Inflammatory Bowel Disease

J.D. Lloyd-Still, Chicago

Factors Involved in Reported Cases of Colonic Strictures

1. Associated with high-strength lipase enzymes (>20000 units).
2. Associated with excessive dosage (>18000 units/kg/meal).
3. Associated with prolonged duration of administration (over 6 months).
4. Associated with age group 2-5 years.
5. Associated with meconium ileus in 50% of cases in the U.S., but not in Europe.
6. Restricted to cystic fibrosis patients.

Personal Experience of Intestinal Strictures in CF

I reviewed our experience of strictures in the intestine, which involves 25 years of looking after over 500 CF patients. Specifically, we have seen 379 CF patients in the last 20 years at The Children's Memorial Hospital in Chicago.

1. Intestinal strictures were seen in 4 CF patients during this time.
2. All these patients had previous operations for meconium ileus.
3. Ages of presentation were 3 months, 1 year, 4 years and 13 years.
4. Only one has been treated with high-dose enzymes in slightly increased dosage (6000 units/kg/meal).
5. All strictures involved the ileocolic region.

Other Data on Colonic Intestinal Strictures in Humans and Animals

Other causes of strictures in the colon in humans and animal models have occurred in the following situations.

1. With potassium thiazide combinations (in the 1960s). Studies in animals showed that this was mainly a risk in the small intestine and was not related to either thiazide or the slow release preparation but was caused by the potassium

chloride. The mechanism by which potassium chloride causes its damage appears to be, sequentially: absorption in high concentration over a short segment of intestine, action upon submucosal and mural veins, causing venous spasm, stasis, submucosal edema and segmental infarction with ulceration and stenosis.

2. Numerous non-steroidal anti-inflammatory drugs cause strictures without having high affinity for the caecum and ascending colon. These have occurred in epidemic form and 9 cases were reported from Switzerland in 1993. Adults with this complication present with abdominal pain and rectal bleeding, but in some cases only non-inflammatory fibrotic diaphragm-like strictures are formed, although there have been other reports of ulceration with acute inflammatory reaction and vasculitis. Animal models are available.

3. There has been a report of diaphragm-like strictures in a bypassed loop of intestine, suggesting that the etiological mechanism is partially through the bloodstream, since there was no luminal contact with the drug in the diverted segment. A form of inflammatory bowel disease has been described in bypass patients and resolves on reattachment. Bacterial overgrowth in the bypassed segment, with production of immune complexes, is thought to be the cause.

Relationship Between CF and Crohn's Disease

Associations between inflammatory bowel disease and cystic fibrosis are common. The incidence of Crohn's disease in cystic fibrosis is 17 times higher than the reported incidence in the general pediatric population. The various mechanisms predisposing CF patients to Crohn's disease have recently been described in detail [3].

Occurrence of Colitis in Non-CF Patients on High Dosage of Pancreatic Enzymes

As far as we are aware, there is no literature on this subject. We have had personal experience of one non-CF patient who presented in 1991 with steatorrhoea (co-efficient of malabsorption 65%). She had previously been diagnosed with diabetes and was known to have pancreatic calcification. Investigation revealed borderline elevated sweat electrolytes (59 and 61 mEq/l) and quite severe malnutrition. She was thought to have pancreatic insufficiency and was started on pancreatic enzymes in a dosage of 16000 units/kg/meal. This had been gradually increased because each time she took the enzymes, her diarrhoea worsened. She developed abdominal pain and rectal bleeding and, six months later, was found to have evidence of colitis on endoscopy. An x-ray revealed thickening of the transverse colon. The colitis was unusual in that it was spotty, with evidence of chronic inflammation. Further investigations revealed that she had coeliac disease, and therefore she was taken off pancreatic enzymes and put on a gluten-free diet. Subsequently, her colitis resolved, although she has continued on 5-ASA compounds. Her parents always believed that the pancreatic enzymes had caused her colitis. When we first saw her in 1991 we had no data on that association.

Experience of Colitis in CF Patients on High-Dose Pancreatic Enzymes who are Pre-Stricture

1. We have had notification of 2 possible patients as a result of a teleconference experience. The first was a 2 year old CF patient in UCLA Davis who had profuse colitis following excessive doses of enzymes; the case history will be submitted at the October CF conference in Orlando. The second was a similar patient at the University of Colorado in Denver, who had widespread colitis after being treated with excessive pancreatic enzyme doses.

2. We have personal experience of 2 patients with similar problems. The first patient had meconium ileus at birth, with resection of 1/3 of intestine and development of short bowel syndrome. At age 4, he developed meconium ileus equivalent with severe pain. He also had evidence of perirectal abscess and, on colonoscopy, had colitis with maximal changes in his caecal area, with crypt abscesses and fibrosis. Since then, he has had a recurrence of obstruction, and upper GI has shown a strictured area in his ileum. The differential diagnosis is between Crohn's and colitis, aggravated by his high dose enzymes (6000 units/kg/meal).

Another 5 year old patient has had evidence of chronic abdominal pain, diarrhoea, and rectal bleeding for the last three years. He also has developed fissures and perirectal lesions. His initial colonoscopy in 1993 showed microscopical evidence of colitis, but was normal endoscopically. He has continued with symptoms and now has abnormal endoscopic findings and histological evidence of increasingly severe colitis. He had been treated with doses of enzyme that were high (6000 u/kg/day) but not excessive.

References

1. Smyth RL, van Velzen D, Smyth AR, et al. (1994) Strictures of ascending colon in cystic fibrosis and high-strength pancreatic enzymes. Lancet 343:85-86
2. Bjarnason I, Peters TJ (1989) Intestinal permeability, non-steroidal anti-inflammatory drug enteropathy and inflammatory bowel disease: an overview. Got Festschrift 22-28
3. Lloyd-Still JD (1994) Crohn's disease and cystic fibrosis. Digestive Diseases and Sciences 39 (4):880-885

Pancreatic Enzymes Supplements: Administration Guidelines at Genoa (Italy) CF Centre

L. Romano, Genoa and C. Romano, Genoa

The Genoa CF Centre, established in the early 1960s, was the first Italian CF centre. Since its foundation, more than 450 patients have been seen. Currently, 209 patients are in follow-up: the mean age of the series is 16.3 years (range 0.3-43 years); 94 patients (45%) are over 18 years.

The overall incidence of pancreatic insufficiency at the Genoa CF centre is 87% (182/209 patients). Isolated steatorrhoea is the most frequent presenting feature in children younger than 2 years (Fig.1). The incidence of pancreatic insufficiency is somewhat higher among younger patients, being 90% in patients younger than 18 years and 84% in older patients. This might be because, generally, the disease is milder and the prognosis better in patients without pancreatic insufficiency, so that more of these survive into adulthood.

Although the incidence of pancreatic insufficiency in our Centre matches the average incidence in Europe, the frequency of the "severe" mutation ΔF508 is only 53%, comparable to the average incidence in Italy [1]. A different genetic background

Fig. 1. Symptoms at diagnosis in 314 patients observed at the Genoa CF Centre in the period 1970–1992. Meconium ileus is excluded. Isolated steatorrhoea represents the more frequent presenting manifestation in children younger than 2 years. The incidence of bronchopulmonary symptoms increases with increasing age at diagnosis

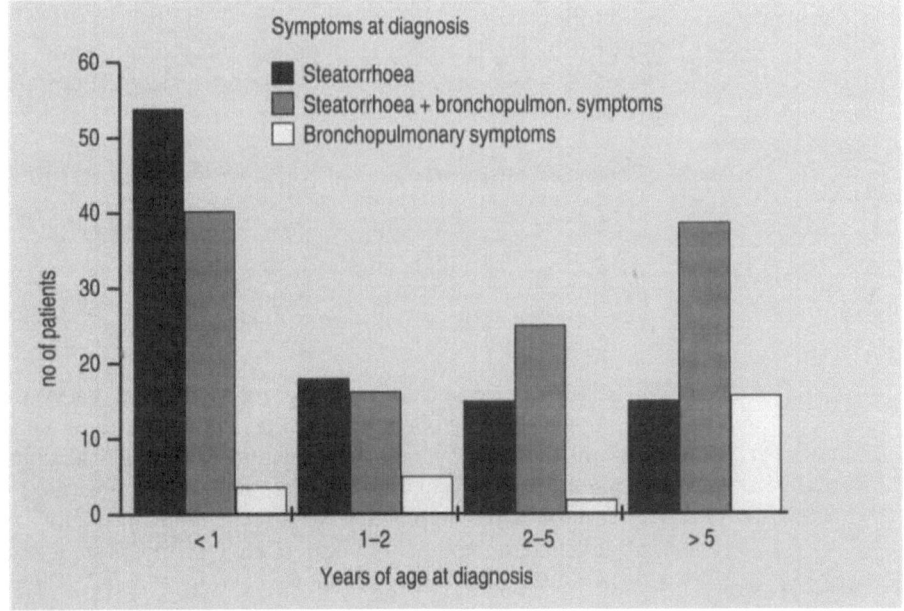

than in northern Europe might partly account for differences in problems with maldigestion/malabsorption control in Italian CF patients. Furthermore, some differences in management may be due to the fact that, of the most common acid-resistant coated enzyme preparations, only Pancrease®-Cilag and Pancrex Duo®-Sandoz were available in Italy until the end of 1993 and no high-strength non-coated powder has been available commercially since 1990.

At our Centre treatment of patients with pancreatic insufficiency with supplements is strictly individualized and it is aimed at improving the clinical picture and symptoms and controlling steatorrhoea.

Patients are instructed to take enzymes at the beginning of each meal, just before or together with the first course. Although the enzyme supplementation, in the form of number of capsules per meal, is prescribed by the CF Centre physician, patients are allowed to vary (by one or two units) the number of capsules according to the size of the meal. When the number of capsules exceeds 6 or 7 per meal, patients are advised to take roughly half the dose at the beginning of the meal and the rest between the first and the second courses.

No particular dietary direction is given at our Centre, but details of food intake are collected every 6-12 months from the patients. The patient (or his/her parent) is asked to record on an appropriate form all food intake during a 3-day period. Foods are registered per meal, so that it is possible to calculate the calories taken in each meal or snack. The patient's diet is analysed by the Dietetics Department and the fat content of the meals is assessed. Whenever appropriate, suggestions are given in order to ensure:

1) an increased caloric intake (ranging from 110 to 150% of recommended daily allowances, according to the degree of pulmonary involvement);
2) a moderately high fat intake (30-40% of daily calories);
3) a normal intake of simple carbohydrates (10% of daily calories).

The number of capsules needed per meal is adjusted according to the fat content of each meal. Presently at our Centre patients receive, on average, approximately 800 lipase units (U.Ph.Eur.) per gram of fat content of each meal (range 600 - 1500 units/g of fat). In practice, when pancreatic insufficiency is established, treatment with pancreatic enzymes is started at a dose of 600 lipase units/g of fat for each meal (Fig.2). Clini-

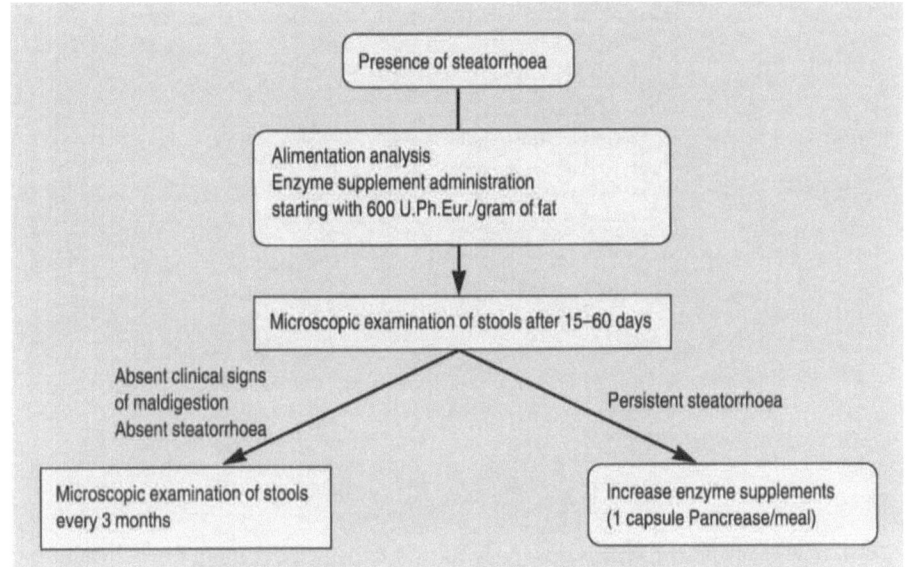

Fig. 2. Flow-chart for maldigestion correction. Genoa CF Centre (part I)

cal status and steatorrhoea are usually re-evaluated 2 weeks to 2 months after the beginning of the treatment. Steatorrhoea is assessed by Sudan III staining and microscopical examination of the stools [2]. Microscopical examination of the stools is a semi-quantitative technique. The test is extremely simple, quick to perform and cheap; the results are immediate and the test can be repeated at each visit. It is also a very rough assay and its use is maybe not sufficiently validated in the literature. Nevertheless, in our experience it has proved satisfactory in routine assessment of the efficacy of enzyme supplementation in CF patients.

When the clinical signs of maldigestion and steatorrhoea on microscopical examination of the stools are absent, enzyme supplementation treatment is considered adequate. Microscopical stool examination is repeated at each visit (generally every 3 months) in children and at least once a year in adults.

If steatorrhoea persists after an adequate period of treatment with supplements, either with or without other clinical signs of maldigestion, the dose of pancreatic enzymes is increased. For practical reasons, the dose is increased by one capsule of Pancrease®-Cilag (that is, by a nominal strength of 5350 lipase units) at every meal. The dose can be further increased after successive periods of treatment if control of maldigestion is considered unsatisfactory by microscopical examination of the stools. If steatorrhoea persists after increasing pancreatic

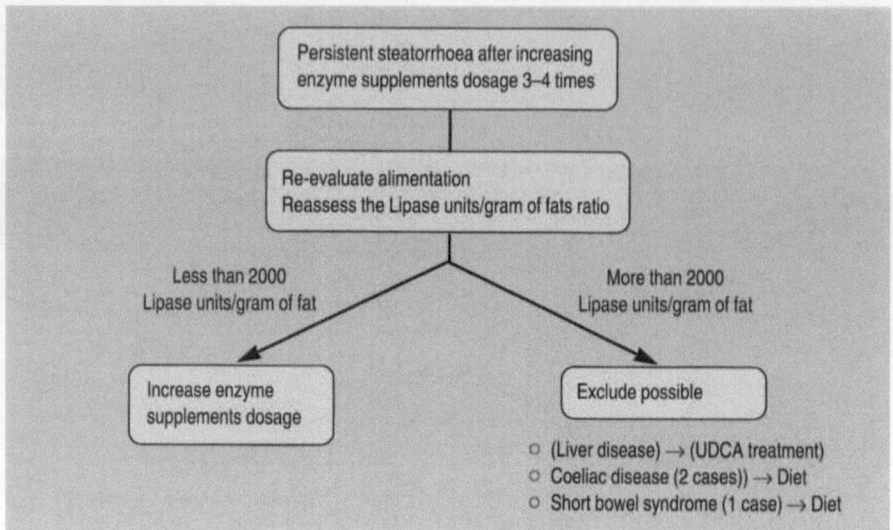

```
┌─────────────────────────────────────┐
│ Persistent steatorrhoea after increasing │
│ enzyme supplements dosage 3–4 times      │
└─────────────────────────────────────┘
                   │
┌─────────────────────────────────────┐
│ Re-evaluate alimentation                 │
│ Reassess the Lipase units/gram of fats ratio │
└─────────────────────────────────────┘
```

Less than 2000
Lipase units/gram of fat

More than 2000
Lipase units/gram of fat

Increase enzyme
supplements dosage

Exclude possible

○ (Liver disease) → (UDCA treatment)
○ Coeliac disease (2 cases)) → Diet
○ Short bowel syndrome (1 case) → Diet

Fig. 3. Flow-chart for maldigestion correction. Genoa CF Centre (part II)

enzymes dosage by 3 or 4 capsules per meal from the starting dose the dietary analysis is repeated, the compliance of the patient to the prescribed treatment is evaluated and the ratio of lipase units/g of fat in the food is reassessed (Fig.3). Further increases in enzyme supplementation are made only if the ratio lipase units/g of fat is below 2000, since we consider that 2000 units of lipase/g of fat in the food is a high dose.

Persistent steatorrhoea despite a high dose of enzyme supplements deserves further investigation in order to exclude possible concomitant causes of steatorrhoea. In particular, attention should be paid to:

1) liver and/or biliary involvement;
2) coeliac disease;
3) short bowel syndrome or malformation.

In our Centre patients are routinely evaluated for liver disease. The prevalence of biliary cirrhosis in our series is 8.4% (on ultrasound scan, with or without portal hypertension). Treatment with ursodeoxycholic acid (UDCA) proved effective in reducing the serum concentrations of liver enzymes and in improving digestion, as evaluated both by fat absorption rate and on clinical grounds [3].

Coeliac disease is relatively common in some countries and appears to be particularly so in some regions of Italy. Although the prevalence of the fortuitous association of the two diseases is expected to be low [4], a higher incidence of coeliac disease in CF patients than in the general population has been

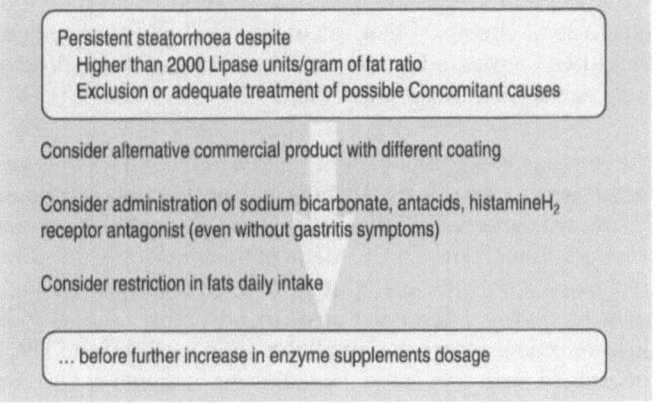

Fig. 4. Flow-chart for maldigestion correction. Genoa CF Centre (part III)

Persistent steatorrhoea despite
  Higher than 2000 Lipase units/gram of fat ratio
  Exclusion or adequate treatment of possible Concomitant causes

Consider alternative commercial product with different coating

Consider administration of sodium bicarbonate, antacids, histamineH$_2$ receptor antagonist (even without gastritis symptoms)

Consider restriction in fats daily intake

... before further increase in enzyme supplements dosage

noticed [5,6]. The hypothesis that CF might predispose to coeliac disease remains unsupported. We diagnosed coeliac disease in three patients with CF (two of them are in follow-up). In all these three patients, steatorrhoea persisted until an appropriate diet was started.

Another patient in our series was diagnosed as having Hirschsprung disease and underwent extensive large-bowel resection. He was on parenteral nutrition for many months until diagnosis of associated CF was made. Pancreatic enzyme supplementation greatly improved his food tolerance and digestion, but he still has short-bowel syndrome and needs a partially semi-elemental diet to control symptoms. This case exemplifies how diseases other than pancreatic insufficiency can account for maldigestion and malabsorption in CF patients, especially when difficulties in controlling steatorrhoea arise.

In a minority of patients steatorrhoea may persist despite the administration of more than 2000 lipase units/g of fat in the food, even when concomitant causes have been excluded or adequately treated (Fig.4). In these patients we consider the option of administration of a different commercial preparation, because pancreatic enzymes with a different acid-resistant coating can sometimes be more effective for a particular patient. A few years ago, patients were changed from various pancreatic enzyme preparations to Pancrease®Cilag because some coatings required too high a pH, so that microspheres were found intact in the stools. In countries where more than one modern pancreatic enzyme preparation is available, a different product should be tried before the dose is further increased. A second choice is represented by the administration of sodium bicarbonate, antacids or a histamine H$_2$-receptor antagonist, even in the absence of gastroduodenal symptoms. Finally, in our opinion, when severe steatorrhoea and/or other malabsorption symptoms persist, restriction of fat intake or even a semi-elemental diet, according to clinical indications, should be considered before a further increase in the dose of enzyme supplements is prescribed.

The frequency of complications related to maldigestion is low in our series. Severe distal intestinal obstruction syndrome (DIOS) was observed in three patients (1.5%): all the patients were adults with known CF. Medical treatment only (rehydration, oral mucolytics, oral gastrografin, enemas) proved sufficient to restore intestinal transit in all cases. Maldigestion proved to be undertreated in all the three patients, and DIOS recurrence was prevented by adjusting enzyme treatment. Crohn's disease may also be associated with unsatisfactory control of maldigestion in CF: two patients in our series (1%) were found to have Crohn's disease. Both were male adolescents, poorly compliant with treatment, and both had inadequate control of maldigestion. One of these patients died shortly after diagnosis of Crohn's disease; the other showed great clinical improvement after achieving a good control of steatorrhoea.

High-strength pancreatic supplements have been recently introduced in Italy. Our preliminary experience shows their clinical effectiveness. Furthermore, it is easy to predict that compliance will be improved if patients can be prescribed fewer capsules.

The administration of high-strength pancreatic supplements has been associated with cases of large-bowel stricture that required surgical intervention [7]. If these strictures are due to high-strength supplements, they might be the consequence of inappropriately high doses, either in absolute terms or relative to the patient's needs. At the doses suggested here, based on the ratio of lipase units/g of fat, the risk of severe complications such as large-bowel stricture should be minimal.

References

1. Ronchetto P et al. (1991) Frequency of cystic fibrosis mutations among Italian patients. In: Tsui LC, Romeo G, Greger R, Gorini S (Eds) The identification of the FC gene: recent progress and new research strategies. Plenum Press Pub New York: 387–390
2. Lelong M, Colin J, Polonowski C (1952) Les stéatorrhées infantiles. Leur charactérisation. Archives Français de Pédiatrie 10: 561–565
3. Cotting J, Lentze M, Reichen J (1989) Ursodeoxycholic acid (UDCA) treatment improves liver disease and nutritional state in Cystic Fibrosis (CF) patients with chronic cholestasis. Gastroenterology 96: A586

4. Goodchild M, Nelson R, Anderson C (1973) Cystic Fibrosis and coeliac disease: coexistence in two children. Arch Dis Child 48: 684–691
5. Park RW, Grand RJ (1981) Gastrointestinal manifestations of Cystic Fibrosis: a review: Gastroenterology 81: 1143–1151
6. Littlewood JM (1992) Gastrointestinal complications in Cystic Fibrosis. Journal of the Royal Society of Medicine. 85 (Suppl. 18): 13–19
7. Smyth RL, van Velzen D, Smyth AR, Lloyd DA, Heaf DP (1994) Strictures of ascending colon in cystic fibrosis and high-strength pancreatic enzymes. The Lancet 343: 85–86

L. Romano, C.J. Taylor, R.I. Smyth and R. Fink

Dr. Romano: Briefly our approach to the problem of maldigestion. First of all the lipase dosage.

The majority of our patients receive approximately 800 lipase units/g fat. Generally, the lipase dose is divided according to the fat content of the meals. Thus an adult taking 4000 calories per day with 40% of the calories as fats will need a maximum daily lipase dose of 250000 - 300000 units.

When steatorrhoea is present we perform an alimentation analysis. Administration of the enzyme supplement starts with about 600 units of lipase/g fat/meal. We also perform microscopical examination of stools routinely in our patients. When enzyme supplementation is first started we usually monitor the steatorrhoea microscopically every 15 or 16 days. When maldigestion is well controlled (no microscopical or clinical evidence of steatorrhoea) the dose is maintained. If steatorrhoea is still present we increase the dose stepwise, adding 1 capsule of pancrease per meal at every increase step.

If steatorrhoea persists after several dose increases the patient's diet is reassessed and the lipase: fat ratio adjusted. If this is less than 2000 lipase units/g fat we increase the enzyme supplement dosage; if it is above 2000 we look for other possible causes: liver disease, coeliac disease, short bowel syndrome and other inflammatory disorders.

Finally, if steatorrhoea persists despite a lipase dose of more than 2000 units/g fat and possible concomitant causes are either excluded or adequately treated, we consider alterative commercial products with different coatings or the administration of antacids, H_2-receptor antagonists or restriction in fat intake before further increasing the enzyme supplements dosage.

Dr. Taylor: I would briefly like to emphasize a couple of the points from the poster that we presented at this meeting giving an evaluation of a high-lipase enzyme preparation in 44 CF patients over two 3-month study periods. In this study we combined subjective assessments (i.e. a weekly diary card completed by the patients) with objective measurements of fat absorption and fat excretion (Shwachman and Crispin Norman Score), lung function and the other parameters that we measure at monthly clinic visits. There was no real difference in the overall condition of the patients or their dietary intake between the two study periods. Neither was there any difference in the terms of growth or weight gain between the two study periods.

Looking at the indices of fat absorption, to get the same amount of fat absorption measured either with an oral fat tolerance test or with faecal fat excretion patients required much more lipase with the high-lipase enzymes than they did with the older preparations. In both arms of the study the majority of patients had normal fat absorption. There were, however, significantly fewer episodes of abdominal pain with the high-lipase preparations. So, our findings are very similar to those presented by Dr. Miller and his colleagues in recent correspondence in the Lancet, in which he showed that patients on high-lipase preparations had less abdominal pain and were less likely to have distal ileal obstruction syndrome. In fact he suggested that the high-lipase preparation may be protective in reducing the incidence of distal ileal obstruction.

I would briefly like to present a case report of a child who presented as a neonate with meconium ileus and was subsequently confirmed as having CF with a Δ F508/508 genotype. He came to our clinic in 1987 aged 7, with a history of persistent malabsorption. At that time he was taking a large dose of standard strength enzymes - at least 70 or more standard-strength Creon a day. He had a good dietary intake with calories and protein 115-120% of recommended daily intake. Despite that he had evidence of a low xylose absorption and a low vitamin A, and he had significant fat loss in his stool. Contrast studies showed a narrowing in the right colon. Jejunal biopsy was normal, and there was no evidence of coeliac disease. He subsequently came to surgery and had a colonic stricture resected. The material from this child was sent to Alder Hey Hospital in Liverpool, where the histological findings were found to be similar to the Liverpool cases. Thus we have a child with a similar stricture, whose pathology antedated the introduction of the high-lipase preparations.

Dr. Fink: I think we need to be careful in interpreting the findings of any studies on enzyme dosage that are not blind, because there is a marked effect of patient preference for taking fewer capsules. Is it just that fewer capsules are associated with fewer intestinal symptoms, or is that a real effect?

Dr. Smyth: I would like to make two or three points from our patients. We have now seen 7 children who have had surgery for strictures. The three points I want to make are (1) about the dose taken and compliance, (2) about the extent of the colonic involvement, which I think in many cases is greater than we first appreciated, and (3) about the association with distal intestinal obstruction syndrome.

Our 6th patient presented at a time when he was on 37000 units of lipase/kg/day. When I went through the notes I found that for a year previously he had been taking a higher dose. On radiology he had what looked like a very short stricture of the ascending colon. In his resection specimen, there was evidence of distension with a wide line of fibrous tissue.

The surgeon said that the operation was very similar to that for Crohn's disease, that he would feel what was normal and join up the two ends. As you know we have had one child with a recurrence from our original series and I am very concerned that that child's remaining colon might not have been entirely normal. We have at least one other in our series who has radiological abnormalities in the remaining colon. I think that this may have been a more extensive process than we first appreciated.

Many of our patients with distal intestinal obstruction syndrome presented with colicky abdominal pain, and we though initially that they had distal intestinal obstruction syndrome, which occurs in fewer than 10% of patients in our clinic. Almost all these children had not previous history of distal intestinal obstruction syndrome, and I think that what they had was not DIOS but a stricture.

Finally, our last patient, a child with evidence of extensive colonic involvements, was also on a higher dose of pancreatic enzymes than was recorded in the notes. This is why in the case-control study that we are now performing we are interviewing the patients and their parents to try to find out precisely what dose they were taking and why and when they changed it.

This patient had a stricture of the ascending colon, with evidence of abnormalities right down. 4 months after the first barium enema and after his ileostomy a further barium enema showed a completely strictured colon down to the rectum.

Discussion

Prof. Dodge: We have heard a lot about the dosage of pancreatic enzymes in cystic fibrosis. I want to raise a cautionary note, and that is that we are dealing with a biological preparation, so dosage is not precise. All manufacturers have the same problem: they are producing a preparation which in the course of time is going to lose its activity, and so they must state the minimum activity that will be available from that preparation guaranteed at the end of its shelflife.

In a paper published this year in the Journal of Clinical Pharmacology the actual enzyme content of pancreatin preparations available in the United States was examined, and the lipase content was found to be between 124% and 155% of the amount stated on the box. How old those preparations were, is not stated, they were probably some time before the end of their shelflife. The protease was 190% of the stated quantity. Thus it is worth bearing in mind that protease is much more stable than lipase, so at the end of the shelflife there would still be 190% of protease with maybe only 100% of the lipase. Thus these patients may be getting a great deal more enzyme than expected.

In our study we used a slightly different method of assessment, and I think that our lipase units are probably higher than those of the manufacturers. One preparation, a product which claimed to have 8000 units of lipase, contained 19000 units (by our method). Thus the high and low strength preparations may overlap in strength, and this might explain why patients transferring from a so-called low-dose or conventional strength preparation to a high-strength preparation will not be able to make a simple arithmetical calculation of dose reduction. It might also explain why some patients prefer one product to another. So dosage, strength and actual content may not be equivalent between products.

Now we have a number of questions. First, what is the best test for monitoring fat absorption? It could be a chemical method, it could be a visual method. Dr. Littlewood made his position very clear. Would any of the other panellists like to comment?

Dr. Fink: For balance studies we tend to use the 72-hour stool fats, but we have found a very good correlation between 72-hour stool fats and what has been called the "steatocrit", which is essentially taking the stool, just a random sample, emulsifying it with an equal volume of distilled water and then spinning it down in a micro centrifuge tube and directly reading the percentage fat. With regard to accuracy, this method has somewhere between a true 72-hour stool fat content and just looking under the microscope, but it appears to be fairly reproducible and is fairly quick and easy to do in the clinic.

Prof. Dodge: Has anyone had experience with the new infrared probes that you simply stick in to a sample of stool?

Dr. Posselt: In Frankfurt we have been using the infrared probe for two years, and the results were published in Gastroenterology about a year ago. There is quite a good correlation between total fat content and the new infrared method. The infrared procedure is quite easy. With this technique we have also measured the stool protein content, water concentration, and so on.

Dr. Taylor: Could I ask those of you who have been doing regular faecal fat studies how that correlates with weight gain and overall control of nutrition?

Dr. Fink: In our clinic we have found that in 95% of patients aged over 25 years the estimation of faecal fats is very useful as an indicator of inadequate nutrition but less useful in indicating inadequate enzyme dosage. Most of our patients who were not growing well had grossly inadequate food intake. So it has shifted our emphasis to looking at daily food intake, putting more effort into nutrition counselling and greater use of high calorie supplements.

Prof. Dodge: I wonder if I could ask the panel some rather more basic questions: do we have an acceptable definition of steatorrhoea or an acceptable one for steatorrhoea at different ages? Dr. Littlewood said that the younger babies seem to require more nutrition. Is that needed more for growth or more to satisfy a predetermined level of fat absorption that we think they should have? And to what extent does steatorrhoea per se matter? Does it correlate with symptoms? Is it a cause of abdominal pain? If it does not interfere with weight gain or weight maintenance and growth, does it matter that a few extra calories are lost? If steatorrhoea is harmful, what is the evidence?

Dr. Littlewood: I think steatorrhoea is harmful because we are always talking about fat, but we do not talk about all the other things - micronutrients, vitamin A, etc. which are lost in the stools. So I think the aim of treatment should be to return the patient to as normal a state as possible. Normal absorption is about 95% of fat as taken in by the mouth, and I think we should be aiming for that. I think we probably achieve over 90% absorption in the majority of patients. We are doing an assessment of other consultants' patients from smaller hospitals, and it is relatively common to see patients with absorption of less than 80%. With this level of malabsorption it is more difficult to achieve the intake needed to sustain good nutrition. We do a 48-hour stool collection over a 7-day faecal marking using a radio-opaque marker. We do not use a steatocrit because we have not found that very helpful.

Prof. Dodge: The dose-response relationship between pancreatic enzymes and fat absorption is not linear, and the dose of enzymes might have to be doubled or trebled to achieve an extra 5% or 10% of absorption. Can we define a cut-off point at which we can say that fat absorption is adequate and we need not increase enzyme doses further unless there is evidence of impaired growth? It would be somewhere between 80%, which I think most people would agree is unacceptably poor fat absorption, and 95%, which Dr. Littlewood is aiming at?

Prof. Lenoir: In my experience children with cystic fibrosis tolerate some types of fat better than others. In France we have used butter, which is not tolerated by young children. I think steatorrhoea is perhaps harmful, but some types of dietary fat are harmful also.

Prof. Dodge: Would you like to tell us how you recommend modifying the diet to reduce saturated fat and perhaps increase unsaturated fat? What do you actually advise?

Prof. Lenoir: I would ask colleagues about the use of semi-elemental diet for babies with CF with about a 50% unsaturated fat content. For babies we regularly use this type of fat without pancreatic extract.

Dr. Littlewood: This is probably an incorrect practice.

Prof. Dodge: Does anyone else recommend using semi-elemental diets routinely in young babies?

Prof. Lloyd-Still: Yes, we do. But I'm not convinced it is the correct thing to do. I think it depends on the age group so much, because the infants are the ones who are so difficult with the caloric intake. I think it was the Milan group who showed that the elemental diet was really good in infants with very severe pancreatic insufficiency. There is a difference between the infant and the older child in terms of absorption.

Prof. Dodge: We have a lady from Milan in the audience. Would you confirm that, or do you think differently?

Dr. Colombo: I don't think the study you're quoting is from Milan, maybe it's from Verona. We monitored the efficiency of fat absorption in infants on a semi-elemental diet and documented an increase in weight gain and a reduction in steatorrhoea. There is a clear correlation between the efficiency of the child's growth and semi-elemental diet.

Dr. Posselt: We have two questions concerning the additional treatment with H_2-blockers and high strength of lipase preparations. Are there any comments?

Dr. Fink: We have routinely added H_2-antagonists to the therapy when patients reach a dose of between 2000 and 3000 units of lipase/kg/meal. I think there may well be a point at which increased enzyme dosage becomes less responsive or ineffective unless the pH of the intestine is corrected. Correcting intestinal pH, whether with an H_2-antagonist or with antacids allows earlier release of enzyme and may thus be very important. I think it is also interesting to point out some observations on the cases of strictures that have occurred. They all appeared to have been in patients taking over 6000 units of lipase/kg/meal, all patients were less than 13 years of age and the majority less than 6 years. As far as I can tell none were on H_2-antagonists. So whether there is a protective factor or not I cannot say. But I think colonic strictures do show more clustering than can be explained by chance.

Dr. Posselt: I think we agree that all the published patients from Copenhagen also had colonic strictures. All of them were on H_2-blockers.

Dr. Steffen: We are discussing the substitution of lipase to improve digestion of fat. Earlier studies showed that lipase is inactivated by acid in the stomach, and this inactivation can be avoided by various means, e.g. by using H_2-blockers, proton pump inhibitors or lipase acid-resistant coatings. All these have certain advantages and disadvantages. The disadvantage of coated preparations is that they slow the release of enzyme into the small intestine. Lipase acts only at the surface of the globules which means that an emulsifying agent such as bile must be present in adequate quantities. So, increasing the dose of lipase might not solve other problems such as inadequate mixing and delayed release. Sometimes the dose has been increased because of inadequate therapeutic response, but this entails an unwanted increase in proteases and amylase as well as lipase. High amylase concentrations give rise to high glucose levels, and high protease levels probably cause side-effects such as perianal skin reddening. So when we speak about dose-related side-effects we should probably think about the dose of protease. When considering therapeutic effects, we should think about lipase dosage, but when considering side-effects we should concentrate on the dose of protease. These considerations have implications for the observed discrepancies between the declared and actual enzyme concentrations in commercial preparations.

Prof. Dodge: We have correlated nitrogen and fat excretion in cystic fibrosis patients. Our experience is different from Dr. Littlewood's because we found that although in general there is a reasonable correlation, some patients have spectacularly higher excretion of fat than nitrogen and vice versa. For the individual patient, good fat absorption does not necessarily imply good protein absorption. Our experience is that the correlation within individual patients is not close, and it is not even consistent between one measurement and another. I think we probably all agree that if pancreatic enzymes are damaging the gut, causing either colitis or strictures, this is more likely to be due to the protease content than the lipase content. Does anyone think that the lipase is likely to be the primary cause of side effects?

Dr. Littlewood: I think it could be. I think we do not know.

Prof. Dodge: I agree, we do not know, but what would be the balance of probability? I would tend to go for protease, but I do not know what other people think.

Dr. Taylor: If you go back into the literature of the development of pancreatic extracts, back to the 1970s when they were looking at a variety of plant proteases, there were reports of gut damage from plant proteases at that time.

Dr. Littlewood: Could I come back to Dr. Fink's point about the H_2-blockers? The introduction of enteric-coated enzymes in the UK resulted in loss of interest in H_2-blockers. In the UK we chose to raise the dose of enzymes, which was better for the patient than having to remember to take an H_2-blocker half an hour before a meal. However, I now like the idea of enzyme-sparing and using H_2-blockers.

I was, however, worried about the long-term effects of powerful H_2-blockers and proton pump depressors in CF patients. What happens to the billions of swallowed organisms that are normally killed by stomach acid, and what is the effect on the normal small bowel flora?

Dr. Fink: I think the reason for using H_2-blockers is not necessarily just to reduce enzyme dosage, but if we are trying to normalize digestion we may need to get a pH that is more suitable for the intestine. The pH of the intestine in CF is much more acidic than normal, so we may be not just releasing the enzyme earlier but giving it to be active in the intestine. That may be an important effect.

Dr. Posselt: What is known about the long term treatment in children? In Germany H_2-blockers are not allowed for long-term treatment in children.

Dr. Littlewood: The pH of the small intestine rises quite rapidly to well over 6 in cystic fibrosis, although duodenal pH may be very low. I think that's quite an important point when you were thinking about release, because certainly these new enzymes are released much lower down the gut. The pH falls rapidly in the caecum but in CF it goes down much more slowly, thus permitting further release of enzyme activity that are down there when they shouldn´t be there.

Prof. Dodge: There has been some other work in adults with chronic pancreatitis showing more or less the same thing, that there is a lot of activated enzyme in the ileum and the caecum. One other approach has been with prostaglandins and there was some quite interesting work from Australia which has been further developed since it was published, which suggests that this might be a very acceptable way to enhance enzyme efficiency, perhaps without the long term theoretical risks of H_2-antagonists.

Prof. Lloyd-Still: We did a double-blind study of prostaglandin, which is not published. We found negative results. There are several problems. One is that it is difficult to give to female patients because of the risk of effects on pregnancy. So it is not very practical for adults. We found great individual variation in effectiveness.
I'd like to make a comment about the H_2-blockers. Reflux is a major problem in all age groups, and H_2-blockers would have a further advantage in helping this. In the 1970s and early 1980s there were reports of strictures of the oesophagus in CF. Some were so severe and so involved that colon interposition was

seriously considered. This was when the old- type enzyme prep-arations were being given, before the enteric-coated prepara-tions.

I would like to raise a possibility. We know these enzymes used to burn the mouth and still do in babies. I suspect that the old enzymes may have burned the oesophagus, and in fact I asked the people in Houston who reported this. I was going to try to get a specimen to see whether there were any character-istics in the oesophagus similar to what we see in the colon with the strictures.

Prof. Dodge: I think you should also take into account the fact that the old-style enzymes would, by their composition, be a very powerful stimulant to gastric acid secretion. It would be a kind of fractional test meal, so you might well be getting a maximal acid response with that amount of raw protein.

Dr. Posselt: We have two questions concerning the change in the gastrointestinal flora caused by antibiotics and so on. One question is: Are there any links between the change in the flo-ra and the strictures? We know that Dr. Koch presented six cases from Copenhagen and he detected *Clostridium difficile* in one of these patients.

Prof. Dodge: I think you can find *Clostridium difficile* in al-most anybody if you look. I took this up with a bacteriologist, who said it depends on what you mean by isolating *Clostridi-um difficile*, and if it was not consistently found in a series it probably was not present in large enough amounts to be im-plicated. Has anyone any factual knowledge or plausible hy-potheses about the role of bacteria?

Prof. Cezard: We have worked on the effects of the antibiotics on the colonic flora, but not in cystic fibrosis patients. We have shown that high concentrations of antibiotics in the co-lon completely destroy the normal flora. That could interfere with the colon. There has been described a lot of transloca-tion, lesion of the colon in very small children because of anti-biotics. The heavy use of antibiotics in cystic fibrosis could be very damaging to the colon.

Dr. Posselt: It might be that the change in the gastrointestinal flora is the first step in injury to the mucosa, with the protease perhaps working later.

Prof. Dodge: I think it is important to remember that the bacte-ria in the colon manufacture short-chain fatty acids, which are an important nutritional substrate for the colon itself. So if elimination of the flora has reduced the supply of nutrients to the gut, then any damage initiated by something else might take longer to heal. In experimental ischaemic bowel damage in animals if you first ligate the pancreatic duct and remove pancreatic enzymes from the picture the lesions heal much more quickly. So there is evidence that pancreatic enzymes naturally produced from the pancreas may actually harm or delay healing in the colon when it has been damaged by some other agent. I think there are a whole lot of variables there, both with the enzymes and perhaps also with the nutrients, that may play a part in producing chronic lesions in the gut.

Dr. Posselt: Is ultrasonography a good way to monitor the gut? How often should it be done?

Prof. Antonelli: In our experience ultrasonography is a good tool to use, especially when we want to study the correlation between enzyme concentrations and dangerous side-effects such as colonic stricture. We had the opportunity to observe thickening of the intestinal wall in four patients who had no sign or symptoms. One of these had wall thickening in the colon. In all patients the thickening reversed very shortly after reduction of the enzyme dose.

Dr. Posselt: That is very surprising if it is a fibrotic change. I do not believe that reversal of thickness is possible after the change of therapy.

Dr. Littlewood: I would just like to make two points. Dr. Smith, a very experienced paediatric radiologist in our hospital, says he does not think that ultrasound is reliable in ruling out early damage to the colon or lack of activity of the colon. Second, I think when you suspect colonic pathology in a patient with cystic fibrosis you should investigate with a barium enema or colonoscopy or you should do a follow-through of contrast medium such as gastrografin, which might give quite a good outline of the colon. I would not rely on ultrasound.

Dr. Posselt: Your pictures of inflammation of the colon were very impressive, but the histology presented from Liverpool showed such a mild degree of inflammation that I do not believe it would be possible to see anything by colonoscopy. Moreover, colonoscopy is quite invasive. We have had a more encouraging experience with sonography. We have seen in some patients a thickening of the submucosa. And in some of these patients had a positive test for occult blood in the stool.

Dr. Littlewood: I've never seen any series of cases looking for occult blood, I don't know whether you have, in cystic fibrosis patients.

Dr. Posselt: It's difficult because you have sometimes haemoptysis and it might be possible by this way. We have to look for it carefully in the future.

Prof. Dodge: How many of your patients are actually anaemic or have evidence of iron deficiency?

Dr. Littlewood: Well, I think less now than when we looked in the past, it might be 15% or something like that.

Dr. Fink: Just a comment on the anaemia. I think there are far more CF patients who have physiological anaemia than we recognize, and if we compare the adolescents and adults with adult models of chronic obstructive pulmonary disease with similar lung dysfunction, CF patients are chronically anaemic. They do not show the reactive rise in haematocrit that you see in chronic obstructive pulmonary disease in adults. It is rare to see a CF patient with a haematocrit of 55 or 60 and yet in an adult lung disease clinic with similar levels of lung dysfunction almost all patients have markedly increased haematocrits. The anaemia is a part of chronic illness because they do not handle iron normally.

Prof. Dodge: Is it iron deficiency or is it protein deficiency and a turnover problem with the production of red blood cells, because they're not only iron deficient, they are also deficient in the protein?

Dr. Fink: It may be more chronic inflammation than iron or protein deficiency.

Prof. Dodge: At what age can we start treatment with pancreatic enzymes? Does anyone think there is any need to delay following diagnosis? No? Well then, what sort of examinations do you do before you start pancreatic enzyme supplementation? Do you need evidence of maldigestion and malabsorption? What would you do in a young infant who is newly diagnosed to confirm pancreatic insufficiency before starting enzymes?

Prof. Antonelli: We measure chymotrypsin in the stools, which is easy and rapid to perform and is a good indicator of pancreatic function. Then we follow with faecal fat content in a 3-day collection.

Prof. Dodge: So you would use stool chymotrypsin followed by faecal fat. Would you do a quantitative faecal fat in a young infant?

Prof. Antonelli: If it is possible to collect the right way.

Prof. Dodge: But not direct microscopy?

Prof. Antonelli: Well, we would consider that.

Prof. Dodge: Has anyone else any different practice?

Dr. Littlewood: I worry that some of these infants are not pancreatic insufficient. I would go along with doing a faecal chymotrypsin and microscopy, looking particularly for neutral fat, and start the baby on a small dose, perhaps one-third of a capsule with each feed at the beginning of feeds.

Prof. Lloyd-Still: We usually do chymotrypsin too, because we do not screen. In one Australian study, 35% of the screened infants had normal function at 6 weeks and about 10% at the end of a year. So clearly this is an evolving disease.

Prof. Dodge: I do not think that a high IRT gives you any indication of what is going out through the pancreatic duct. It tells you what is being absorbed into the bloodstream. I do not think it gives an indication of pancreatic insufficiency until it falls too low to be measured. Then you know that the pancreas has stopped working.

Prof. Lloyd-Still: I am talking not about a screened baby but about one who presents with pancreatic insufficiency at about 4 months of age. I would think that is much more indicative.

Prof. Dodge: Well, what can it mean? It means that there is something wrong with the pancreas.

Dr. Lloyd-Still: It means there is chronic pancreatitis, and I think that is a warning sign.

Prof. Dodge: But it does not mean that the pancreas is not secreting enough enzyme.

Prof. Lloyd-Still: No, I did not say that. I said that I would use it as a warning sign. If the child was growing normally and the stool trypsin was normal we would not automatically put him or her on enzymes.

Dr. Romano: I would like to comment on microscopical examination of the stools, because steatorrhoea must be massive in order to be informative by this method, especially in the first weeks of life, when even normal babies show neutral fat droplets in the stools

Dr. Littlewood: I think we must go back to clinical examination, because in many of these babies, even the screened ones, the diagnosis is not confirmed until age 4 - 6 weeks, by which time a good proportion of them will be not thriving and will have a slightly distended abdomen and obviously abnormal stools. In those circumstances if we then find a low chymotrypsin and a lot of neutral fat we would start enzymes, because you can always withdraw them and think again. The point is to get the baby thriving.

Prof. Lenoir: Do we all agree that a baby born with meconium ileus has a pancreatic insufficiency?

Prof. Dodge: No, I think Shwachman showed about 25 years ago that some babies with meconium ileus had adequate pancreatic function. Whether they subsequently became pancreatic insufficient I do not know, and I do not think he ever published that. But he showed that they had a functioning pancreas at birth.

Prof. Dodge: Do abdominal symptoms reflect the degree of malabsorption?

Dr. Fink: Our experience has been that abdominal symptoms correlate very poorly with measured steatorrhoea at least. It is important how you ask the question. If you tell patients their stool is normal they assume their everyday pattern is normal. So you have to ask specific questions. But even so I think there is a very poor correlation. In a study on enzyme dosing we found many patients who had abdominal symptoms and greater than 90% absorption of fats. Their symptoms did not appear to be related to steatorrhoea. Increasing enzymes on the basis of abdominal symptoms such as cramping or pain can lead to difficulties.

Prof. Dodge: What about stool odour? It is related of course to protein maldigestion and not to fat maldigestion, so if the stools smell offensive that suggests that protein absorption is inadequate and as I have said earlier protein absorption might not correlate very well with fat absorption. When patients say they are better on a particular preparation it may be because it contains more protease.

Prof. Lenoir: In the study of Peter Durie, faecal fat in 240 treated CF patients from Toronto was estimated. One third had less than 10% malabsorption, a third had 10 - 20% and a third had 20 - 50%. I discussed this with Peter, because there are a lot of patients who have steatorrhoea above 20 g (up to 75 g) a day without any abdominal pain or other symptoms. These are patients who do not receive high-dose enzyme supplements and have a normal growth curve.

Prof. Lloyd-Still: How does this fit in with Dr. Littlewood's data?

Dr. Littlewood: It fits in perfectly well. Our record holder was a 30-year old man who had no complaints at all and was passing 170 g of fat a day in his stools. He thought that was normal. I agree that in the individual case there is a very poor correlation between symptoms and steatorrhoea. However, if you look at a population of 300 patients complaining of symptoms then I think you will get a correlation with steatorrhoea and complaints of symptoms. What patients complain of is very subjective. You might have a non-complaining patient with severe steatorrhoea who is asked in the clinic "Are your bowels alright?" and the answer is "Fine".

Prof. Lloyd-Still: I thought you said 90% of your patients had excellent absorption. Dr. Lenard said 30% do not. Is that correct? So there's a 20% difference?

Dr. Littlewood: Well I think absorption in Leeds is probably better than in Toronto.

Prof. Lloyd-Still: That's what I'm trying to bring out. Which makes it even more interesting because they claim that their growth and everything else are wonderful. It is all related to nutrition, but when it is shown that a third of patients are not actually absorbing, that makes me wonder whether it is only a question of absorption.

Dr. Littlewood: They are big eaters.

Prof. Lenoir: This could be the difference between what children or young patients eat in North America and in Europe.

Prof. Dodge: No, because Peter Durie said yesterday that there was no need to give very high intakes, that his patients were managing very well on 110% of the recommended daily allowance. Dr. Littlewood´s are all taking between 120% and 150% and getting 90% fat absorption, so whether they are any bigger or any better than the ones in Toronto remains to be seen.

Dr. Littlewood: They are smaller than Canadians, so we force them to get bigger.

Prof. Lenoir: I think they eat more fat than we do in Europe.

Dr. Littlewood: What percentage of their intake is fat, I wonder, because it is difficult to get over 40%, I think. I don't know, maybe someone disagrees.

Dr. Taylor: Prof. Dodge, you will recall the data from the study comparing Toronto and Boston in terms of growth and survival. Would you know what percentage of patients were pancreatic sufficient?

Prof. Dodge: Well, I think that's a very important point because the Toronto clinic claims that up to 15% of its patients are pancreatic sufficient. This is certainly not the experience of any clinic I know of in Europe, and I doubt whether it is the experience in Boston either. All of which is very intriguing.

Prof. Lloyd-Still: I do not think the correlation between pain and steatorrhoea is at all good. In fact Kevin Gaskin when talking about liver disease makes the point that all the patients with liver disease have pain. That is how they recognize them, and they have a huge number of patients with liver disease. So I went over all our patients trying to find out whether our patients with liver disease had pain. I could not find that kind of correlation. That is another question I should like to ask. Is it the experience of the panel here that the patients with liver disease have a higher frequency of pain than the patients without liver disease?

Dr. Colombo: Our experience is that the frequency of abdominal pain is not higher in patients with liver disease. We have a lot of patients with meconium ileus equivalent in the liver disease group. The abdominal pain is often related to distal intestinal obstructions. So our experience does not agree with Gaskin's.

Prof. Dodge: Well, Gaskin's patients with liver disease all had strictures of the bile duct too, so again I prefer that we do not go down that particular road this afternoon.
Can we come back to a question about high dosage, because I think we need to get towards our consensus if we can. In Germany only 7% of patients receive more than 20000 lipase

units/kg body weight/day. What were the reasons for these high doses? Professor Posselt, do you know why this group of patients had very high doses?

Dr. Posselt: We do not have exact data for all our patients, but I know that Dr. Stern in Tübingen looks very carefully at fat excretion and monitors patients up to a high dosage. But certainly we have to discuss whether giving large doses of enzymes is a good way to increase fat absorption unless adjunctive treatment, e.g. with H_2-blockers, is given too. I do not know exactly why many other centres give high dosages. Some of the younger patients from Frankfurt are not monitored by fat excretion at present, more by the feeling of the parents and the doctors. I think it's quite dangerous.

Prof. Dodge: We will now move toward our consensus. Could I ask Prof. Posselt if he will give us a review of the suggested therapeutic guidelines.

Dr. Posselt: In patients in whom malnutrition and maldigestion are difficult to control we have to exclude infections of the gastrointestinal tract, other diseases such as coeliac disease, sugar intolerance and food intolerance, inflammatory bowel diseases and anatomical abnormalities. Oesophagitis has been mentioned, and the metabolic changes of diabetes, which can lead to malnutrition, must, I think, be carefully looked for. Liver cirrhosis and portal hypertension can lead to malnutrition, and I think it is very important, too, to exclude psychological problems and behavioural feeding difficulties. Many of these problems are common in younger patients, and I think over-protection from the parents is one of the biggest problems in this field.

Guidelines to exclude failure to thrive:

1) We have to pay more attention to educating parents and patients, to teaching them good feeding habits and telling them what percentages of fat are in different kinds of food.
2) We have to adjust the energy intake to an age- and disease-related normal intake.
3) We then have to adjust pancreatic enzyme supplementation to food intake and to decide whether H_2-blockers, and perhaps bile salts, are also needed.
4) We have to be sure that the patients are compliant and we have to exclude other disorders, related or not related to the cystic fibrosis.
5) We have to optimize the treatment of lung manifestations in these patients and evaluate them for psychological problems and start interventions if necessary.
6) In addition, we have to decide which patient needs nutritional supplements

With respect to the observed **colonic strictures**, we have to train the patients in feeding habits. We have to choose the best type of preparation for the patients, and from today's discussion this seems to mean taking a low-dose lipase preparation for as long as is acceptable. We have to inform patients about the correct intake of enzymes, to tell them perhaps to take half of the suggested dose at the beginning of the meal and half during the meal if their appetite is good. Then we have to make sure the patients are compliant with treatment.

Perhaps a dose of 15 000 or 20 000 lipase units/kg body weight/day is a little too high. In Germany at the present time 15 000 units is the accepted upper limit. Perhaps it is better to calculate this on the basis of grammes of fat intake. In addition, we have discussed H_2-blockers, but we have not discussed the increased use of MCTs in the very few patients in whom maldigestion is uncontrollable by other means. Further, we should perform laboratory controls to avoid strictures by regular stool fat excretion, monitor compliance by measuring chymotrypsin in the stool, and perhaps we should look for occult blood in the stool and, with regular ultrasonography, examine the thickness of the bowel wall. We have not discussed the problems we encounter in patients treated with H_2-blocker. We know that Cisapride increases gastric emptying and intestinal transit, and it is possible that the amount of active enzyme in the ileum and caecum are increased with this treatment. Many patients with meconium ileus equivalent are treated with Cisapride today.

Guidelines for medication with pancreatic enzymes are:

1) The dosage should be adjusted to the suggested food intake.
2) The total amount of enzymes should be divided over the whole course of meal, i.e. the first portion should be taken at the beginning of the meal, the second depending on the total amount of food intake (i.e. appetite) at the end (Dr. Littlewood: The second half should be taken later in the middle of the meal).
3) If the capsules are opened, the microtablets should be given with juice, tea or water, i.e. not with a fluid with an alkaline pH.
4) Combined medication with drugs accelerating gastric emptying and GI transit might be harmful.
5) Self-dose regulation is not allowed without prior consultation with the physician in charge.

Prof. Dodge: I think you were saying that we should regularly monitor for thickening of the bowel wall. Are you suggesting we should do that even in patients who have no symptoms or only in those who have abdominal pain or evidence of colonic abnormalities?

Dr. Posselt: I think at the present time we should do it as a prospective study in a bigger group of centres, yes.

Prof. Dodge: As an investigation rather than a regular part of management?

Dr. Posselt: As an investigation at the present time, perhaps maintaining treatment with high-lipase preparations for all patients.

Prof. Lloyd-Still: How many meals a day do your patients get in Germany?

Dr. Posselt: Five.

Prof. Lloyd-Still: That answers my question, because one of my questions was: can there be consensus to relate dosage of enzymes to units of lipase/kg/day or kg/meal? I think that is important because in the US we have been taught to do it with every meal, yet people there eat snacks throughout the day and this is a very difficult problem. This might well double their requirement for lipase - some eat eight times a day.

Dr. Posselt: The problem is that if we calculate this on the basis of grammes of fat intake/day, we have to ask them to record their intake, which is a bit difficult. It is easier for daily management to calculate it on the basis of kg body weight.

Dr. Dabardie: Did you notice any side effects?

Dr. Posselt: I have no experience of side effects with respect to the strictures, and this is something we must discuss.

Dr. Taylor: My own feeling is that your limit of 15 000–20 000 is too low. Most of our patients, certainly our younger ones, would need more than that. Also, we have talked about using H_2-blockers and yet I am not aware of convincing evidence that H_2-blockers actually work in CF. The best study I know of showed that although H_2-blockers enhanced the effectiveness of conventional enteric coated preparations they had no effect on the microsphere preparations. In our experience a very large dose of a proton pump blocker is needed to get the pH up to about 5.

Prof. Dodge: But are you trying to get your pH up or are you trying to improve your fat absorption?

Dr. Taylor: Well, one should follow the other.

Prof. Dodge: It should, but it may not necessarily, like everything else in CF.

Dr. Taylor: You can certainly see that in the first couple of hours after a meal the pH is rarely above 4 in many patients.

Prof. Lenoir: I agree with much of Dr. Posselt's strategy, but I wonder about two points. The first is that fat malabsorption is difficult to analyse and has perhaps nothing to do with action of the pancreatic extract. I have some doubt about efficacy. The second point is that the addition of another drug is proposed if pancreatic extract causes side effects. I do not understand this point, because the obvious first response is surely to reduce the dose of the pancreatic extract and perhaps not to add any drug, because we know nothing about the interactions with other drugs. Antibiotics are necessary in cystic fibrosis, but H_2-blockers? I do not know.

Dr. Posselt: I think I mentioned that it might be harmful to use Cisapride. Treatment with H_2-blockers might be an asset to reduce the pancreatic enzymes, but I have had problems with long-term treatment with H_2-blockers in children.

Prof. Cezard: I would like to comment on the proposition about faecal fat estimation. What is important, I think is, for us not to prescribe high doses of pancreatic enzyme. If the child is growing well, faecal fat does not matter very much. This has been shown in many studies. Faecal fat is important but not essential. What is essential is normal growth. That should be the principal criterion, rather than faecal fat. If faecal fat is high but growth normal I think it is not necessary to increase the pancreatic enzyme. If there are symptoms, we should look for another cause in case it is not the pancreatic insufficiency that causes the steatorrhoea.

Dr. Littlewood: I do not agree with that.

Prof. Dodge: Clearly this is one point on which we are probably not going to reach a consensus today.

I was asked to summarize the meeting. I worked on some questions earlier in the discussion about things that I thought we might be able to agree on. First, at what age can we start treatment with enzymes? Well, I think there's general agreement that if there is evidence of steatorrhoea, and there may be different ways of obtaining that, then treatment should be started at the time of diagnosis. If not, the patient should be monitored for evidence of malabsorption.

Secondly, is there any evidence that high-strength lipase preparations pose a special problem related to their formulation, or are any possible side effects attributable to the high total dose of enzymes? It is obviously more difficult to achieve very high doses with lower-strength preparations, but Dr. Taylor's one patient who had taken spectacularly large numbers of capsules suggests that that may be the problem, that it is the high total dosage rather than the strength of the capsule that matters.

Thirdly, can we define an upper limit of safety for dosage? Dr. Fink suggested that no strictures had occurred in patients receiving less than 6000 units of lipase/kg/meal, suggesting that that might be a possible upper limit of safety. But he also quoted Lebenthal´s proposal, which I think is probably generally accepted in the US, that normally we should say about 3000 units/kg/meal, which translates in American terms into about 15 000 units/day. This is exactly the same dosage that the Germans arrived at, bearing in mind that some patients have a kind of grazing intake rather than one of regular meals. I agree with the proposal that if we can relate the lipase intake to the diet and to the fat content of the diet, that is probably the best thing to do. Professor Romano showed us how that can be done. This has also been a suggestion from Germany.

Another question I asked myself is: when should we be satisfied with the level of fat absorption achieved? Here there is a divergence of opinion. We have heard from Prof. Lenoir indirectly that Peter Durie believes that we should be guided by clinical parameters, so that if the patient is doing well we may tolerate a degree of steatorrhoea, which would perhaps not be acceptable to everyone. I think Dr. Littlewood would feel happier if we managed at least 90% fat absorption. I think there is work to be done in that area, to define acceptability. We would all agree that anything below 80% is totally unacceptable unless the patient is doing extremely well. It seems that some of Peter Durie patients are in that category, but I would not be happy with a fat absorption of less than 80%, and I do not suppose most of us would. 85% I might accept, Dr. Littlewood would press for a bit more. So I think we need to do some work in that area to define whether and when we should add adjuncts such as H_2-antagonists or prostaglandins. If we suspect that there may be side effects in the form of colonic pathology, how should we investigate it? We have discussed ultrasound, contrast enemas and occult blood, and the proposal is that, at least for the near future, we should regularly examine the colons of our patients by ultrasound and perhaps by occult blood.

The last question, which I do not expect to be answered today, is: is there within the CF population a susceptible sub-group of patients perhaps with an altered intestinal flora? No one has asked whether something like a relative deficiency of alpha-1-protease inhibitor is a factor. Is there a group of patients with a particular genotype who may be more susceptible to the action of exogenous protease? I do not know, but I think it might be worth asking, and that is a testable hypothesis because we could look at their genotypes and their alpha-1-protease levels in blood, which we assume reflects what happens in tissue.